REBEL HEALTH

REBEL HEALTH

A Field Guide to the Patient-Led Revolution in Medical Care

SUSANNAH FOX

The MIT Press
Cambridge, Massachusetts
London, England

The MIT Press would like to thank the anonymous peer reviewers who provided comments on drafts of this book. The generous work of academic experts is essential for establishing the authority and quality of our publications. We acknowledge with gratitude the contributions of these otherwise uncredited readers.

This book was set in Adobe Garamond and Berthold Akzidenz Grotesk by Jen Jackowitz. Printed and bound in the United States of America.

Library of Congress Cataloging-in-Publication Data

Names: Fox, Susannah, author.
Title: Rebel health : a field guide to the patient-led revolution in
   medical care / Susannah Fox.
Description: Cambridge, Massachusetts : The MIT Press, [2024] | Includes
   bibliographical references and index.
Identifiers: LCCN 2023013906 (print) | LCCN 2023013907 (ebook) |
   ISBN 9780262048897 (hardcover) | ISBN 9780262378079 (epub) |
   ISBN 9780262378062 (pdf)
Subjects: MESH: Patient Participation | Professional–Patient Relations |
   Patient Advocacy | Quality Assurance, Health Care
Classification: LCC R727.42 (print) | LCC R727.42 (ebook) | NLM W 85 |
   DDC 610.696—dc23/eng/20230912
LC record available at https://lccn.loc.gov/2023013906
LC ebook record available at https://lccn.loc.gov/2023013907

10 9 8 7 6 5 4 3 2 1

For Eric, for everything.

Contents

Preface

Why *Rebel Health*?

Rebels are creative, independent, and action-oriented. They bend rules and make their own tools to change the world for the better. For more than twenty years, I have collected stories and evidence from rebels on the front lines of an underground movement to improve health and health care. This is a revolution you will want to join.

Everyone who feels forgotten or lost in the shadows of suffering, whether navigating a new diagnosis or life with a chronic condition: you are not alone. Expert networks of patients, survivors, and caregivers stand ready to help. I will show you how to find them.

Rebel Health is also for anyone working inside health care who is fed up with the status quo. It is a competitive advantage to partner with the people who are closest to the problems you are trying to solve. I will give you new strategies and ideas for how to approach your work.

I wrote this book in memory of Tom Ferguson, MD, who urged me to spend time in online patient communities starting in 2001. Pioneers were building the missing infrastructure of health care, weaving a net of information, data, and tools to save themselves and anyone else who needed help. They were joined by forward-thinking clinicians, funders, executives, and government leaders who saw the value of working with patients, survivors, and caregivers. But there is still so much to do.

Join the patient-led revolution. Together we can heal health care.

1 SEEKER, NETWORKER, SOLVER, CHAMPION

Dana Lewis is a very deep sleeper whose alarm often failed to wake her up. She was not anxious about being late to her job as a digital media strategist. She had bigger concerns: dying in her sleep.

Lewis lives with insulin-requiring diabetes. In 2013, she worried that the alarm for the device that monitors her blood sugar was not loud enough to rouse her, especially if her levels went low in the middle of the night. One of the most common causes of death from diabetes is nocturnal hypoglycemia or "dead in bed" syndrome. Lewis could go to sleep with her blood sugar in a healthy range, not sense that it was dipping to dangerous levels, and never wake up.

Lewis, who lived alone in Seattle, and her mother, back home in Alabama, worked out a system of early morning calls and texts to be sure that Lewis woke up every morning, safe and sound. But Lewis wanted independence. Why should her mother have to continue to worry about her? Lewis wrote to diabetes device manufacturers, asking them to make louder alarms. Their answer? No. The alarms are loud enough. They didn't seem to care that the alarms weren't loud enough for Lewis or any of the other deep sleepers in their customer base. In shutting her down, device makers ignored the possibility that they could learn from one of their users and improve their product.

Before the internet, before peer-to-peer connections among people with the same condition became easier, Lewis may have given up. But she did not.

Lewis knew she could build a custom alarm if only she could get access to her continuous glucose monitor (CGM) data. Luckily, she is part of an online community of people living with diabetes.

In February 2013, a software engineer in upstate New York named John Costik tweeted about how he had been able to free the data from his four-year-old's CGM. He was part of an underground rebel alliance of people who were tinkering with diabetes devices, reverse-engineering their software and communication protocols, and then sharing what they found. With the community's encouragement, Costik publicly shared the details of what he'd done and, within days, Lewis replicated his methodology to get access to her own device data.

She devised a working alarm that was loud enough to wake her up, which she then shared online. That continuous cycle of knowledge-sharing and experimentation places Lewis, Costik, and other problem-solvers on the front lines of the patient-led revolution, where their questions are being answered and their needs are being met, often independently from the mainstream health-care system. This revolution is the start of something big—for them and for all of us. And like all revolutions, its roots are deep and it has many organizers.

DEEP ROOTS

People have always learned from each other, person to person, outside of formal institutions. Historically, neighbors, friends, and family members were each other's first responders, second opinions, and collaborators. People who were isolated or shut out of medical and research institutions bravely created their own.

Rapid advancements in drug development and clinical training in the last 100 years has extended and saved countless lives, even as it changed the landscape of American life. Consider the changes we have seen at the start and end of life:

- In 1900, 95 percent of births happened at home. Nowadays, nearly every birth in the United States (98 percent) occurs in a hospital.
- In 1949, half of the deaths in the United States occurred in institutions like hospitals and nursing homes. By 1980, that percentage rose to 74 percent of deaths. Death at home has surged in the last decade, however,

surpassing hospital deaths for the first time since the early twentieth century.

The good news is that science has mostly won out over unproven remedies and unsafe practices. The bad news is that professionalization sidelined outside innovators and lay health experts. Health care was taken out of the home, out of the hands of family members and community helpers. Scientific exploration and publication expanded past the ability of any one person to keep up with advancements. For example, in 1976, seven hundred medical journals were circulating in the United States. There are now about thirty thousand medical journals indexed by the US National Library of Medicine.

But the new model of professional health care does not serve everyone's needs. If someone's questions are not visible and interesting to scientists, then doctors are not likely to have any treatments to offer. Discrimination kept Black people and immigrants out of treatment centers into the late twentieth century and even today, their needs go unmet. Unethical researchers conducted notorious experiments on Black people and other vulnerable groups without their consent, further exacerbating unequal access to care and information. Shame or stigma prevents others from speaking up or they are not believed when they do tell their stories. Rare diseases go begging for research funding. .

Those with nowhere else to go turn to each other. They set about gathering or creating the materials, resources, and information they need. They share what they find with wider circles of people, and together, they refine their ideas and practices.

Our human need for connection is tenacious. History shows that you can't stop people from finding—or creating—what they need to solve a problem for themselves or a loved one, despite barriers and scarce resources. Community is a superpower.

A TIME LINE OF PEER-LED HEALTH MOVEMENTS

1867: The United Order of Tents is founded by two formerly enslaved women to provide health, social, and financial assistance to Black people.

1920: Black Cross Nurses is founded to train lay health workers to provide first aid and nutrition counseling to the Black community, which was not being served well under "medical Jim Crow."[1]

1935: Alcoholics Anonymous (AA) is founded as a peer-to-peer mentoring group that guides people to take their sobriety one day at a time.

1948: Fountain House is founded by a group of people with serious mental illness to reduce the social isolation experienced by themselves and their peers.

1953: Narcotics Anonymous is founded, following AA's peer-led model.

1956: La Leche League is formed as a peer mentoring program for those who want to breastfeed their infants, which many doctors discouraged at the time.

1963: Weight Watchers is founded, based on a model of in-person meetings and peer support for weight loss.

1970: Boston Women's Health Book Collective publishes peer-led research about birth control, childbirth, abortion, and menopause (which later becomes the bestselling book, *Our Bodies, Ourselves*).

1971: The Black Panther Party creates a peer-led initiative to test Black people for sickle cell anemia, a genetic disease that is found predominately in people of African descent.

1972: The Berkeley Center for Independent Living is founded as a peer-led community organization for people with disabilities.

1983: Catholic nuns and other volunteers begin MHP Salud, a peer health program for farmworkers and their families that recruited people from the local community as the educators or "promotores."

1983: Living Through Cancer, a forerunner of both the National Coalition of Cancer Survivorship *and* Survivorship in Indian Country is founded to help cancer survivors connect with each other.

1983: People with AIDS write the Denver Principles, demanding fair treatment, respect, and autonomy.

1992: Members of the AIDS Coalition to Unleash Power (ACT UP) form a separate nonprofit to push pharmaceutical companies and the federal government to develop and test therapies for HIV.

IMPACT

Each of those organizations made a significant contribution to pre-internet, peer-led health movements and to American society. Grassroots leaders made progress in areas abandoned by the mainstream health-care system.

For example, AA is one of the most effective—and least expensive—programs available for helping people with alcohol use disorder to moderate or quit drinking altogether.

Rates of breastfeeding in the United States climbed thanks in large part to La Leche League's peer-to-peer advocacy. In the 1950s, just one in five babies was breastfed. Now, four out of five babies born in the United States are breastfed from the start, lowering their risk of obesity, asthma, diabetes, and ear infections, as well as lowering their mothers' risk of high blood pressure, diabetes, ovarian cancer, and breast cancer.

Weight Watchers, when measured against other interventions in population studies, has proved to be a cost-effective model for achieving and maintaining a healthy weight.

A Black Panther Party volunteer, Mary T. Bassett, realized the supply of tests for sickle cell anemia was outstripped by the need and asked Bill Wallace, a biology graduate student, for help. Wallace created a homemade test with elements that volunteers could mix up each week, at low cost—an advance spurred by a peer-led, radical health movement.[2]

Thanks to the awareness brought by the Black Panther Party's innovative data collection effort, $500,000 was allocated to sickle cell anemia research in the National Sickle Cell Anemia Control Act of 1972—a pittance, but a start.[3] The Black Panthers also fused scientific and medical expertise with lay wisdom to create a network of clinics and health workers who could deliver care where and when people needed it.

Ed Roberts, a founder of the Berkeley disability rights coalition, helped lead the movement to deinstitutionalize people with disabilities across the United States. Instead of seeing disability as a medical problem to be fixed, the independent living model reframes it as an opportunity for community learning and support.

MHP Salud now serves as the primary health provider in some of the most isolated and vulnerable Latino communities in Florida, Michigan, Ohio, Texas, and Washington.

Eleven years after the founding of the National Coalition for Cancer Survivorship, its advocacy led to the establishment of the Office of Cancer Survivorship at the National Cancer Institute (NCI) in Washington, DC.

By forming peer-led coalitions, educating themselves, and establishing their credibility, ACT UP and its allies won over scientists and policymakers, creating a partnership that fundamentally changed biomedical research practices.[4]

I ended the history time line in the 1990s because that is when the internet began to go mainstream, helping radical health movements to scale up more quickly than ever before. Online, people are able to share ideas, solve one piece of a health problem, and fit it into a bigger—and more public—puzzle.

Today's rebels stand on the shoulders of these remarkable leaders. And peer-led organizations are poised to dramatically expand the reach of their work.

REBEL HEALTH

My life's work has been to explore and map the terrain created by patients, survivors, and caregivers. While at the Pew Research Center and then as an independent researcher, I spent time in online health communities and conducted national surveys to measure the scope and impact of the patient-led revolution. As the chief technology officer at the US Department of Health and Human Services (HHS), I acted as an ambassador between the worlds of technology, innovation, and health care, and gained a view of these trends at scale. The world has changed in extraordinary ways because of the internet, but I will show that it has the potential to change even more as more people discover that the real power of technology is to connect us not only with information but also with each other.

That change can't happen soon enough. Health care in the United States is broken and expensive. My focus is, and always has been, to open up access to information, data, and tools so people can make better decisions and solve their own problems.

After working at the intersection of technology and health care for more than two decades, here's what I see:

The internet has transformed industry after industry, but health care remains maddeningly immune, characterized by clipboards, fax machines, and retro software. A patient dropped into the existing system is carried along, as if on a conveyor belt, with little information about how they might improve their outcomes. Information flows around them and is collected from them, but rarely are they asked to contribute ideas about the devices, treatments, and services they use.

We all turn to the internet to search for answers. "Dr. Google" is the de facto second opinion for many. Social media platforms are full of people sharing their stories, asking questions, but the chances of finding the right information at the right time are low. Studies show that people are likely to trust a peer's recommendation of a business or service, rating the information that fellow consumers provide as more credible than what a business leader or journalist might say. We crave connection with someone who has faced the same decisions or endured the same symptoms—a "just-in-time someone-like-you." But most people don't know how to begin to look for fellow patients and caregivers who can advise them. There is no systematic way to find help. Too many patients and caregivers feel alone in their struggle.

Meantime, health care is ripe for transformation. We need all the ingenuity we can get to untangle and improve it. But we are leaving half the team on the bench: patients, survivors, and caregivers. And they are primed to get in the game.

We need to take what we have learned from the exchange of information that happens on platforms like Reddit, Facebook, and Wikipedia; mix it with what we know already works in medicine; and unleash the potential of the rebel health alliance. We need to take these unrecognized experts seriously precisely because their influence is so much more important than in other sectors. Our health is at stake.

It may reassure you to remember that peer-to-peer learning is standard in medicine. Clinicians attend conferences and read journals in their specialties, trading insider knowledge about the latest treatments and procedures. Researchers and clinicians who solve a puzzle are likely to share the answer, particularly if they have a platform to do so. In some exceptional clinical centers, patients and caregivers work in partnership with clinicians and researchers, tapping into a pool of specialized knowledge and adding their observations to the evidence base.

But most patients, survivors, and caregivers who track and share their observations are not trained researchers. They do not attend professional meetings. But they blog. And they tweet. And they post on Facebook, YouTube, and in online communities, creating shadow peer-to-peer learning networks that have real benefits for the few who know about them. Some of the most valuable health insights come from anecdotes: What does a heart attack, childbirth, or dialysis really feel like? How do you shower with a leg cast—or help a loved one with dementia bathe safely?

Patients are also teaching each other how to conduct research, to safely experiment, and to ask better questions. Expert networks of patients, survivors, and caregivers have grown up between the cracks of the health-care system. We need to tap into their wisdom, learn their ways, and give fuel to the rebel alliance that is building up our collective capacity for better health.

This book is a field guide to the revolution. Like everything related to health, it is a human story, and I hope it will inspire you to think about your own life, your own family, and your own community.

I met self-care advocate Tom Ferguson, MD, in 2001, and he encouraged me to talk directly with online health pioneers. I now have more than twenty years of notes based on interviews and surveys of a wide range of patients, survivors, and caregivers living with both rare and common health conditions. This book draws from that fieldwork, as well as from the deep well of other scholars' work in the emerging fields of digital health and participatory medicine. All the people I write about are real, and only one person appears under a pseudonym—"Edwin Murphy" in chapter 3.

These true stories expose a cornucopia of opportunities for clinicians, policymakers, investors, entrepreneurs, and anyone else interested in improving health outcomes.

On a personal level, anyone who wants to navigate the health-care maze faster will want to become a health rebel or recruit some to their team. You never know when a new diagnosis or crisis will upend your plans to stay on the sidelines of health care. That's why one audience for this book is the general public.

On a systemic level, it is a competitive advantage to understand and leverage the power of connection among patients, survivors, and caregivers. Tips for entrepreneurs, clinicians, policymakers, investors, and other business leaders are highlighted throughout since they are among the people I hope to inspire.

Mainstream health care needs to invite the rebels inside. We need to connect these out-of-the-box thinkers with the resources they need to test and scale their ideas. This book lights the way forward.

PEER-TO-PEER HEALTH CARE

The word "peer" expresses a state of equality and partnership. Peers, in the context of this book, share symptoms, diagnoses, genetic variants, and lived experiences. Peers pool resources and, when they are given a gift, they pay it forward. They know things about themselves and their bodies that, when shared, are valuable to others with similar challenges—and, as I will show, to all of us.

In 2011, about a decade into my exploration of health and technology, I coined the phrase "peer-to-peer health care." I was alluding to peer-to-peer computing, a distributed network architecture that allows every connection to share resources with its mates, equally and directly. The traditional model of health care centralized power and information, like the old client/server network architecture. People had to go through an intermediary, like a clinician, to access health information. The internet exploded that system and flattened the hierarchy, allowing people to connect directly with information and with each other.

At the same time as these technological changes, it became fashionable to describe health-care services as "patient-centered" (rather than physician-centered, the default setting). Clinicians invited patients to learn more about their diagnoses and participate in treatment decision-making.

The people you'll meet in this book are more radical. They do not wait to be invited. They seize opportunities to take action. They reject the menu of options being offered and instead cook up their own solutions, together. They are rebels: mission-driven, optimistic, and creative.

We have the opportunity to catch up to these pioneers and to get them the resources they need to do their work, which benefits all of us. They are currently working outside the system, but it does not have to stay that way. Innovators should not have to scrounge for resources and materials.

In writing this field guide, I documented and named four archetypes: Seeker, Networker, Solver, and Champion. They are defined more by what they do than who they are since people can take on different roles at different times whether they are patients, caregivers, clinicians, policymakers, or business leaders. Here's a brief description of each so you can start looking for them:

SEEKER

Seekers sense that something is not right with their health and decide to take action. Maybe a diagnosis has dropped them into a maze filled with new terms and treatment options. Maybe their symptoms are mysterious, their worries are deep, and clinicians are not able to answer their questions. Seekers set to work, often hopeful but also often angry and frustrated.

Seekers go out on the hunt.

NETWORKER

"You are not alone." People who are newly diagnosed or facing a health challenge long to hear those words. Connection is an antidote to suffering and confusion. When they are able to tap into peer-to-peer networks of patients and caregivers, Networkers learn in community about their condition, cast off the burdens of isolation and shame, then urge each other to stand up for themselves. Networkers pick up signals and, if we tune in and listen, they can serve as an early warning system for crises—and solutions.

Networkers pool resources.

SOLVER

Solvers identify challenges, then test and develop new concepts, codes, and inventions to meet their needs. They work on a problem with a singular focus because their life—or the life of a loved one—often depends on their ability to invent a solution. They creatively get access to what they need, bending and sometimes breaking rules in pursuit of a goal. Some Solvers openly share their designs online for other people to build on. Others keep their cards close to their vests, working inside regulatory and corporate structures.

Solvers attack problems.

CHAMPION

Champions help take scrappy new ideas to scale. They give Seekers, Networkers, and Solvers access to resources held by mainstream institutions such as funding, media attention, regulatory guidance, or access to labs and manufacturing facilities. They make connections and see opportunities that others miss.

Champions fast-track innovations.

AN ECOSYSTEM OF INNOVATION

Seekers, Networkers, Solvers, and Champions fuel an ecosystem of rebel health innovation. Without peer-to-peer networks boosting the signal for worthy new ideas, inventions languish, never getting noticed or tested. Businesses go unbuilt, and people who would benefit don't learn of a solution to their problem.

I call this book a rebel health field guide because I want readers to be able to spot examples of each archetype "in the wild." When you meet a Seeker, notice how they pursue answers to questions and consider how you can learn along with them. A Networker can connect you with people and resources that are otherwise unrecognized. Solvers are an asset to any team, as they attack problems in creative ways. Recruit them to your cause. Follow Champions to see where opportunities are ripe. Being able to see each of these rebels for the value they create is an asset whether you seek personal or systemic progress.

I highlight stories of patients and families facing unusual health challenges because the study of rare diseases often yields breakthrough insights that benefit those with common conditions. If we create a health-care system that serves these exceptional people, it will serve everyone.

You will also read about people who took shocking chances, experimenting on themselves or tinkering with the devices that keep them alive. Others post their most personal health details online in the hopes of finding people who share their plight. They represent the radical leaders of an underground movement to open up biomedical innovation. I applaud their bravery and ingenuity, but I do not recommend all their methods. Be inspired, but please be cautious. Talk with a clinician before embarking on any new treatments.

Chronic conditions are also featured characters in this book because health is something that can be built—and broken down—quietly, without the fast-moving drama of a life-changing diagnosis. You will meet people living with treatable conditions, as well as those who have not yet—and may never—find a cure.

I call this a patient-led revolution but I also shine a spotlight on caregivers. They are the parents, partners, children, friends, and other loved ones whose work undergirds our health-care system. Caregivers, along with patients and survivors, are an untapped resource, full of ideas for how to improve every aspect of care.

I did not have space to cover the cost of health care in the United States, but it is another frontier of the patient-led revolution since it relates directly to access and availability of treatments and devices.

PROSOCIAL, NOT ANTI-SCIENCE

Everyone featured in this book is prosocial, not anti-science. They have transitioned between or combined the roles of Seeker, Solver, Networker, or Champion, using every tool they can find to change their fates. Their stories include a wide range of peer health communities, those that are purely patient-led and others that are staffed by trained moderators and health professionals.

The ability to connect with people you may never meet in person is one of the opportunities of the internet age. You can follow their stories, share your own, and trade observations on every imaginable topic. But when it comes to online health information, there is an elephant in the room: the danger of misinformation.

Misinformation about vaccine safety is the number one concern associated with peer-to-peer health advice—and for good reason. Anti-vaccine voices are very loud on social platforms, and they have been wickedly effective at grabbing the attention of people who are hesitant about immunizing themselves or their children. The COVID-19 pandemic increased the volume—and the risk—of misinformation to a fever pitch.

However, most parents in the United States vaccinate their children on time. They listen to clinicians and don't fall into the traps laid for them by anti-science activists. And we should not discard the tool of peer connection before looking for ways to make its use safe.

In one study looking at the risk of misinformation, researchers reviewed two years' worth of messages posted to an online patient community focused on implanted cardiac defibrillator (ICD) treatment. They found that half of the advice shared was benign or helpful, one-quarter of the material shared was incorrect, and 6 percent was controversial. That's sobering. But, overall, the study found that the message board provided "a succinct, accessible, and well-organized resource of basic information of interest to ICD patients and candidates" that "may provide a reliable reference to which providers can refer patients."[5] Similar studies have been conducted among other patient populations with equally heartening results.

Clinicians do not have the time—and in many cases, they lack the lived experience—to counsel patients and caregivers living with complex health conditions. Peer patients are filling in the gaps, connecting online and offline, providing advice to help those who are newly diagnosed and unsure about how to handle their next step.

For some, the absence of authority figures in their peer health community is a plus. They don't want the "white coats" sticking their noses into every conversation. They only want to hear from people who have walked the same path.

Other people prefer professional guidance. They want to know there are guardrails and chaperones, people who will step in if the conversation veers toward misinformation or abuse. Because even if online communities self-regulate over time, as studies show, newcomers may enter the conversation and, at that moment, see a post that contains false information. The echo chamber of algorithms compounds the danger.

Instead of trying to shut down patient-led conversations, telling people not to go online, and driving them underground, there should be stable, safe platforms with fact-checking guides and other resources. We need to tip the playing field in favor of truth and give people the tools they need to defend themselves against falsehood. The fact is people always—and will always—turn to each other when they need help.

RIPE FOR INVESTMENT

In addition to gathering stories about health care, I have included lessons learned from user-driven innovation in other industries, both in the United States and abroad. What sounds new and risky in a health context is a tried-and-true technique in designing sports gear, financial services, equipment for space exploration, and online shopping experiences.

I also include tips for readers who aspire to be Seekers, Networkers, Solvers, or Champions gleaned from my interviews with people who have successfully traveled those paths. Those pointers appear in boxes throughout the book, as do summaries or "takeaways" at the end of each chapter.

This book will help you spot patterns in the landscape, both pitfalls and opportunities, as the rebel health flywheel starts to spin faster in the years to come. As a patient or caregiver, you will want to tap into these resources. As a policymaker or business leader, peer-to-peer health care is a problem-solving tool that will help you unravel some of your biggest challenges.

I am offering a new way to understand the full picture of suffering and potential for improvement in the health care system. There are markets ripe for investment out there. A deep reservoir of energy and invention is waiting for us. Let me be your guide. Come along, dive in, and see what I see.

Takeaways:

1. People connect to face health challenges together. The internet enables new problem-solving capabilities and accelerates the patient-led revolution.
2. There is an ecosystem of health innovation powered by Seekers, Networkers, Solvers, and Champions.
3. Misinformation and disinformation are significant threats. We need to boost the signal for prosocial, pro-science messages.

2 SEEKERS

When Burt Minow was born in 1922, his disability—partial hearing loss and complete facial paralysis—was immediately apparent. His mouth was frozen in a sort of frown, and he could not drink like a typical baby. Doctors advised his parents to put him in an institution and forget about him.

But his mother had an indomitable spirit. His parents took him home, found a way to feed him, and raised him alongside his younger siblings. When it was time for Burt to go to school, his mother forced the school system to take him, confident that he could handle the work despite his limitations. He succeeded, eventually graduated from college, and enjoyed a long career in the family laundry and dry cleaning business in Milwaukee, Wisconsin. His niece, Nell Minow, recalls that her Uncle Burt "was dearly loved by all of us for his witty poems and loyalty to underdogs of all kinds, especially the Chicago Cubs."

Unfortunately, few people outside his family attempted to communicate with Burt. He couldn't move his lips when he spoke, so talking with him was like talking with a ventriloquist. And it was difficult to get used to looking at someone whose facial expression never changed.

Because Burt's condition was so rare, it was not until many years later that he even had a name for it: Moebius syndrome. It is a neurological condition affecting the sixth and seventh cranial nerves, which control a person's ability to smile, blink, suck, and move their eyes side to side. For some people, it affects the form of their hands and feet, requiring surgery or other interventions.

When Nell began using the internet in the mid-1980s, she realized that if her uncle went online, he could finally have relationships that were not limited by his disabilities. She set him up with an account, and he began communicating with people who shared his affection for the soap opera *Days of Our Lives*. On the screen, represented only by text, Burt's wit could shine.

A few years later, as the web developed, Nell tested new search engines by typing in arcane terms just to see what came up.

One day she got a hit on a search for "Moebius syndrome." A family with a young child with Moebius had created a website and located hundreds of people around the world with the same diagnosis.

When Nell emailed them about her Uncle Burt, they immediately wrote back, asking his age. At the time, the medical literature was quite limited and had no record of anyone with Moebius living past their thirties. For all they knew, that was what they could expect for their child. When Nell wrote back that Burt was in his seventies, the family rejoiced and started spreading the word.

That day, hundreds of families heard, for the first time, that their loved ones could have a typical life span. And Burt Minow heard, for the first time, that there were other people like him.

As Nell says, "For the last year of his life, he was the elder statesman of a very small but very excited community, and it would not have been possible without the web."

HOPE IS AS VALUABLE AS A CURE

People with Moebius are an extreme example of a common challenge: to find people who share the same concerns, frustrations, and hopes for a better way of doing things. This extremely rare condition—affecting fewer than one in 300,000 or even one in a million by some estimates—has no known cause or cure. Before the internet, people like Burt Minow were unlikely to ever connect with someone else with Moebius. They and other people with rare conditions were completely alone in their struggle.

"But rare isn't so rare when there are one hundred of you," says Natalie Abbott, who lives with the condition, when describing an in-person

Moebius conference. "Instead of hope for a cure, for me and others with incurable conditions, hope is the state of mind fostered by a strong community who knows and accepts the fact that not all things in life can be cured. Hope comes through connections, resources, strength, and time, instead of in a pill. But hope is as valuable as a cure."

This chapter is about Seekers, who embody hope and action. They try one more search term, call one more clinician, or reach out to one more friend for help. Like Nell Minow, they are often acting as proxies for a loved one. Like Abbott, they may be looking for community, not a cure. The health care system works best if everyone facing a challenge either has a Seeker on their team or becomes one themselves. Seekers go out on the hunt.

QUICK ANSWERS TO BURNING QUESTIONS

It's easy to see why people with unusual health challenges need to search online to find each other. But a condition doesn't have to be rare for a community of peers to be useful. Those with more common conditions also benefit from firsthand guides. Chronic conditions such as diabetes, heart disease, and stroke affect six in ten US adults. Many spend hours trying to find each other online to ask questions and exchange ideas—or to simply say, "I'm here. I see you." Many more should, since peer connections could help them, but do not know how to begin.

Think about the four in ten adults in the United States (ages 18–59) who live with human papillomavirus (HPV). Chlamydia, gonorrhea, syphilis, HIV, and other sexually transmitted infections and diseases (STIs or STDs) are less prevalent but still affect millions of Americans. Imagine how each person represented in those statistics worried, wondering if that rash, burning sensation, or blemish was something they should get checked out.

Some go online for advice and ask each other.

On Reddit, a social platform that hosts conversations about a seemingly infinite range of topics, one community, /r/STD, is devoted to information about sexually transmitted diseases. A study published in the *Journal of the American Medical Association* included an analysis of those posts:[1]

- Nearly 17,000 posts were written on /r/STD between 2010 and 2019.
- Eighty-seven percent of posts requesting a crowd diagnosis received a reply.
- Median time for a first response: three hours.

Do these statistics seem outlandish? A quick, personalized response is what people have come to expect from their online communities.

Whether users have a lifelong condition like Moebius or a (hopefully) temporary issue like a treatable infection, the internet enables peer-to-peer connection.

SEEKERS QUESTION

Everyone feels alone at some point in their health journey. Seekers do something about it. If you are a patient or caregiver, channel that energy. If you want to see change happen on the front lines of health care, help people become Seekers. They are the spark that ignites progress.

At first, Seekers are all questions, no answers. They represent frustration and unmet needs. Maybe they are embarrassed about their symptoms. Maybe they don't yet have anyone to turn to. Maybe they don't even know how to accurately describe what's wrong. Maybe they can't afford the time or cost of seeing a clinician. Maybe they are not using health care in a way that can be easily tracked and analyzed—and therefore their needs are invisible to public health agencies, which could help. The 3 a.m. Dr. Google consult is a classic Seeker activity.

Then: a connection.

Think of a time when you have found one other person like you, one other human being who can say, "I've been there too." This is a magic moment! It can happen online or offline, out in the open, or behind a screen name, and, even if it lasts only for a moment, it can change your path. Together, you can pool your knowledge and navigate the health care maze more speedily and more safely. Who benefits? Everyone: patients, caregivers, and all those who want to improve health outcomes. If you are a leader of an organization that cares for or includes people living with chronic conditions, encourage them to become Seekers, to ask questions, and to look for alternatives.

SEEKERS OFTEN—BUT NOT ALWAYS—BECOME NETWORKERS

The Moebius group and the /r/STD group illustrate different ways some Seekers gather and become Networkers. One is a long-term and well-established community, while the other is relatively ephemeral. Both rely on social platforms to disseminate their work. For every one person who is able to travel to the biennial Moebius meeting, there are many who will follow the social media updates or read about it later online. For every one person brave enough to post their question to /r/STD, there are many who are silently monitoring the conversation. They, too, discover they are not alone in seeking answers to uncomfortable questions. They learn where they can find answers when they need them—and maybe advise friends who are in the same situation. Connection to useful information and to each other is their experience and, in time, their expectation.

But not every Seeker will be inclined to join or create a community. They want information, not support. They want to solve a problem they face and move on. They work alone and do not want to compare notes with other people with the same condition. Their discoveries and solutions are lost to the rest of us. If this describes you, please try to find a way to share what you learn for the benefit of other people like you. We need your insights.

SEEKERS ARE VULNERABLE

There are still people who do not go online, some not by choice. In the United States, a significant portion of people living in rural and tribal regions are cut off from high-speed internet access. Even if they do go online, many cannot find answers to their questions. Four groups are particularly vulnerable:

- those with undiagnosed conditions;
- those who carry shame or embarrassment about their health condition;
- those who feel invisible or alone; and
- those who don't know how to begin.

Seekers are often highly motivated to find someone—anyone—who understands what is going on, but they may find it extremely difficult to do so. The next section is about how Seekers can begin to feel their way forward in the dark maze of health care.

SEEKERS DO NOT GIVE UP

Some people can't describe their symptoms in ways that a clinician can understand. They walk out of a clinic empty-handed or with an incomplete diagnosis that describes just one symptom, like "eczema" or "nonspecific, low-back pain." Or patients are given a vague catchall diagnosis, which is essentially the doctor saying, "I don't know what this is, but here's what I'm calling it for now." Chronic fatigue syndrome is one example of this phenomenon, now upgraded to a more scientific term—myalgic encephalomyelitis—and gaining recognition as a post-viral illness. Another example is the slang term "fascinoma"—a mysterious collection of tumors and symptoms.

Worse, a clinician may dismiss someone's symptoms, implying that they indicate a vaguely-specified mental health issue instead of pursuing a meaningful diagnosis. Or patients can't find help that fits into their cultural or social context. People go online to look for the answers that clinicians can't or won't provide.

If you are nodding your head in recognition, you are—or have been—a Seeker. Seekers reject the unsatisfactory answers being offered. They show

---

Tip for Seekers: Learn How to Tell Your Story

Capture the basic elements of your health story so far in a list, an essay, a series of charts or drawings—whatever helps you get started. Gather all the details you can: gene variants, symptoms, diagnoses (even the incorrect ones), and treatments that you have tried (whether they have worked or not). Think about what is most meaningful and important to you. Emphasize those aspects. Then, when you need to, you can tell your story in a useful, coherent way.

courage in the face of isolation, worry, and doubt. They do not give up until they get what they need.

A PG-13 DIAGNOSIS

Another vulnerable group is Seekers who are embarrassed or ashamed of their condition. Peers bridge the gap when you can't work up the courage to tell your friends and family what you have.

Brett Alder was the picture of health at age twenty-four when he married his college sweetheart. During their honeymoon in Mexico, Alder began to have flu-like symptoms—fatigue, muscle soreness, and an inability to concentrate. He thought he had picked up a bug while traveling, but when the symptoms persisted, he started to wonder what else had changed in his life recently that could be causing his illness. The only significant change that he could think of is that he had become sexually active. As a devout Mormon, Alder had abstained from all sexual activity prior to his marriage, including masturbation.

When they returned home to California, he and his wife started tracking his symptoms and found that they were episodic. Immediately after sex, he would get a headache, sore muscles, and throbbing nerves. The day after, his brain felt foggy, and he had trouble concentrating. They moderated their sexual activity to see if that made a difference and were able to isolate the trigger: Alder would have symptoms for seven days post-ejaculation.

He searched online, using the phrase "male allergy to sex," and not only did he not find any relevant results, but Google suggested an alternative search: "Did you mean *male addiction to sex?*"

After six months of reactions, Alder was in a state of chronic pain, and he could no longer use a computer mouse with his right hand because of repetitive nerve damage. He tried to seek medical attention but couldn't get anyone to take him seriously. After describing his symptoms of illness after sex, the first general practitioner simply blinked and deadpanned, "You look perfectly healthy. I don't expect I'll be seeing you often." When he saw a rheumatologist, the doctor listened carefully but only wrote down "myalgia," or muscle pain, in his chart. Another specialist told him that his condition "didn't make sense" and left it at that. Alder was astounded that his description of the problem seemed to carry no weight.

For seven years, Alder suffered in silence, not sharing his health problems with anyone besides his wife and his best friend. He continued to search online for clues but found very few. He once saw a story online about a man with similar symptoms, but when Alder reached out to him via email, the man never responded.

In 2011, Alder once more turned to Google. This time he was elated to find a research paper describing his condition. Researchers in the Netherlands had conducted a study of forty-five men who were allergic to their own semen. That's when Alder learned the name of his condition: post-orgasmic illness syndrome (POIS).[2]

The paper described Alder's symptoms: thirty minutes after ejaculation, allergic reactions involving the head, eyes, nose, throat, and muscles would begin. All forty-five men in the study reported those internal symptoms—the most important evidence when diagnosing an allergy. Thirty-three of them consented to a standard "skin-prick test," which can serve as a secondary confirmation. The procedure is to inject a small amount of an allergen—in this case, the men's own semen—into their forearms and watch for any reaction. If a red, swollen bump appears within thirty minutes at the test site, a true allergy is present. Most, but not all, of the men in the study had a positive skin-prick test.

Armed now with evidence, Alder found an allergist willing to administer the test. But when the doctor administered the injection, they did not see the red, raised bump that would indicate an allergy. Sitting in the exam room, Alder described a strong internal reaction to the injection—and would be sick for the next seven days—but the allergist refused to confirm the diagnosis. After dismissing Alder's wife from the room, the allergist asked if perhaps he had guilty feelings about sex and if this were some type of avoidance behavior. Alder was speechless.

He now had what he calls his "PG-13 condition name" and the knowledge that exposure to his own semen appeared to be the root cause of his ailment. Using more exact search terms, he finally connected with a small group of fellow sufferers online. He joined the online forum and began following the conversation among people who, for the most part, hid their identities but shared crucial information about how they were living with this condition.

Alder went public with his condition when announcing a peer-to-peer health start-up he cofounded. Reflecting on his experience, he said, "When there's no place for you in the medical industry, or you go to join an online community, but can't because you don't know the name for your condition, you feel like there's something wrong with you. As iPhone designer Jonathan Ive has said, 'When our tools are broken, we feel broken.' I was done feeling broken."

Alder's story is one of a Seeker who thought they would never find another person like them, who was told that their problem was mental, not physical. If you blush even thinking about your symptoms or are daunted by the health challenges you face, be brave. Share your worries with a trusted friend. Look for a way to share your story—or search for others—that feels safe, including anonymously.

MISSED OPPORTUNITIES

In the early days of the internet, medical professionals saw online communication as yet another opportunity to educate, but not to listen. They wanted to control the flow of information and, of course, it would only flow one way,

---

Tip for Seekers: Pick a Proxy

You may feel overwhelmed. Or squeamish. Or fearful. You may want the benefits of being a Seeker, but you are not ready to dive into the research yourself. Ask a friend to be your proxy. They will join the relevant communities, search using key words and hashtags, ask your questions, and sift through all the answers. This is a great role for someone who wants to help but who lives far away.

Think about what you want to know ("How quickly do I need to start treatment?") as well as what you are not yet ready to see or hear (for example, surgery videos or worst-case scenarios). Your proxy can gather all the information and insights for you to read at your own pace.

---

from clinicians to patients. Professionals were not asking patients what they wanted to learn, much less contemplating what wisdom they—the clinicians—could gather from communities of people living with a disease or disability.

In her book, *Studying Those Who Study Us*, Diana Forsythe describes how, in the 1990s, she conducted fieldwork in an artificial intelligence lab that was asked to create an information kiosk for newly diagnosed migraine patients.[3] The idea was that patients could walk up to the kiosk, punch in questions, and get information about their condition before or after they saw their doctor. The project was ahead of its time in some ways. Clinicians wanted to give patients in their waiting rooms a chance to educate themselves. But when it launched, it was a failure. Patients told reviewers that the kiosk was not useful. Why? As Forsythe writes, "The research team simply assumed that what patients wanted to know about migraine was what neurologists want to explain."

The kiosk failed to answer the number one question among people newly diagnosed with migraine: am I going to die from this pain? It's an irrelevant, even silly question from the viewpoint of a neurologist, but it is a real fear for people who are in severe pain.

The developers had neglected to talk to any patients. They relied on an interview with a single doctor to tell them what he thought patients should want to know. They also believed the myth that while patients had much to learn from their neurologists, the clinicians had nothing at all to learn from their patients. The developers missed their chance to create a resource that not only had a spigot for dispensing information but also an intake valve for patient observations and contributions.

One of my mentors, Tom Ferguson, MD, shared a memory of a conversation he had with Forsythe, who said, "In practice, most medicine is ten parts culture to every one part real science. And from a medical anthropologist's point of view, a good deal of what happens in the health care system we've all grown up with is invisible to most clinicians. Imagine that."

NEEDS NOT MET

For years I have tried to find ways to explain the particular challenges facing those with undiagnosed or rare health conditions. Or all the people whose treatments are painful, unpleasant, time-consuming, or a burden on their loved ones. They wish for ways to make their situations better. They often have useful ideas for improving their care. But they are not yet connected to each other and are unable to share what they know to benefit others.

Now add all those people who are caring for a loved one, by some estimates four in ten US adults, who have been thrust into a role that they have not been trained for, like managing complex medications at home or performing maintenance on home health equipment.

Think of everyone who is newly diagnosed, whether it is for something low-stakes or serious, who wishes they could find a just-in-time someone-like-them.

There are also, unfortunately, millions of people who can't afford their medications or otherwise do not have access to the care they need. They could benefit from being connected to a peer group to help them navigate the health-care maze.

All of a sudden we are talking about a massive group of people whose health-care needs are not being met by the current system. Their questions are not being answered. We need to recognize such groups more quickly than we have in the past. Here is a visualization that can help (figure 2.1).

Needs not met ———————————————————————— **Needs met**

Figure 2.1
Needs spectrum.

Imagine a horizontal line. On the far left side are the people whose needs are not being met. Their questions are not being answered—or even explored—by scientists and clinicians. Friends and family may not know or understand what is going on. They are totally alone and at sea. At the right are those whose needs *are* being met by the current health-care system.

Central to this model is that people get to decide if their needs are met and their questions are answered. It is not for the rest of us to say. If a remedy or explanation does not work for someone, even if it works for a majority of people, then that person's needs are not met. We must listen to the people in pain, the people who are suffering, the people with doubts. As Dave deBronkart, a patient advocate, told me, "Patients have more at stake than anyone else in determining whether health care is getting the job done for them. Omitting the ultimate stakeholder from running the system and monitoring its success is a fundamental design flaw."

For example, if the best treatment for your condition comes in the form of a pill that is too big for you to comfortably swallow—or too small for your trembling hand to manage—then your needs are not being met. If you have doubts about the options being offered and nobody is willing to answer your questions, then you are also likely on the needs not met side of the spectrum. And, of course, if you cannot afford the device or drug that would solve your problem, then no, your needs are not being met (figure 2.2).

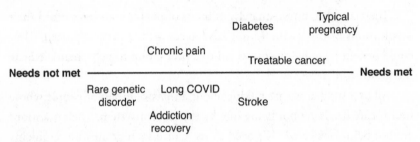

Figure 2.2
Needs spectrum with examples.

At the far right of that horizontal line are the people whose needs *are* being met. Their questions have been answered to their satisfaction. They have a diagnosis. There is not only a range of treatments available but scientists are working diligently on formulating new, better ones. Let's go out to the far end of the spectrum, where people in this segment of the population can both tolerate and afford the treatments offered—and the therapies work. A cure or other resolution is at hand. Maybe their health condition is even something that is celebrated, like a healthy pregnancy and uncomplicated birth. Good for them!

But what about all those people who are not being well-served? Once you start looking, you will see that there is a significant, anguished group of people gathering online. Some of them are too stunned, exhausted, or in despair to take action. Some do not yet know there is an alternative to accepting the status quo. We need to help them become Seekers, who go out on the hunt for something better.

Takeaways:

1. Seekers are a massive group of people with unmet health needs. This is both a crisis and a market opportunity.
2. Isolation is dangerous. Connection is a survival tactic.
3. Peers offer crucial firsthand advice and emotional nourishment that cannot be found elsewhere. Together, they can start to solve problems.

3 TACTICS AND COURAGE

Delina Pryce McPhaull's brother-in-law has a tremor due to Parkinson's disease. Unfortunately, one of the pills he has to take is so tiny that it can easily bounce off the table and disappear. As she wrote to me, "Every time he has to take it, he drops it. It is tiny and, well, he has Parkinson's. I can't tell you how many times the kids end up on the floor looking for the pill he just dropped. Are there any hacks for a Parkinson's patient to manage those tiny pills?"

Pryce McPhaull used the word "hack" in its original sense: an appropriate application of ingenuity. She is a Seeker. She knew that I was collecting examples of "home health hacks"—ways that people were repurposing or modifying everyday objects to solve a problem—and figured I could connect her with a broader community of people who are solving challenges in a creative way. She was right.

I posted her question on my blog and on Twitter, two of the platforms I use to gather and share ideas about navigating health and health care. Within a few days, a half-dozen people weighed in with suggestions, like putting honey or applesauce on a spoon so the pills stay put. Others described how to repurpose dispensers meant for other tiny objects, like artificial sweetener tablets or seeds. One person wrote that they live with cystic fibrosis and must track tablets that seem unnecessarily small: "I have tried to take it up with the company that makes the pills but they have zero interest."

None of the solutions was perfect. Nobody knew of a pill dispenser that fit the bill. But the comments keep rolling in, week after week, year after year. People's needs are not being met by the current system so, as Seekers, they search online for possible solutions. Some of them stumble upon my blog. They are grateful to have found a trading post for ideas and add their own workarounds before moving on.

This chapter is about what Seekers need as they go out on the hunt and how the rest of us can help them.

SEEKERS NEED PEOPLE TO TUNE IN

There is often a mismatch between what mainstream health care wants to build and the problems that patients need to solve.[1] Pharmaceutical companies keep making tiny pills for people living with tremors or low dexterity. Medical device companies and health systems hoard data about people's own bodies. Researchers prioritize work that will land them the academic endorsement that comes from publication in a prestigious journal rather than solving everyday challenges. They ignore—or do not even see—the issues that crowd the left side of the needs not met spectrum.

People living with chronic diseases, by contrast, manage a wide range of daily tasks and note gaps in clinicians' understanding of their condition, usually on their own and with little professional training or support. Their workarounds—or unanswered questions—are a deep well of potential products, services, and research projects. Seekers expose health-care gaps every day. Everyone else needs to tune in, learn from them, and help them.

For example, people living with Parkinson's disease (PD) told investigators that, in addition to pursuing a cure, they would prioritize research that would help them maintain their balance, prevent falls, improve their sleep and urinary function, deal better with stress and anxiety, stave off dementia and cognitive decline, better understand medication side effects, and monitor their specific experience of living with PD.[2]

But these patients' top concerns have not yet been prioritized by researchers. Patient-led networks can shine a light on the path forward by organizing and agitating for change. What new assistive device or therapy could be created to help with fall prevention, for example? Or solve another dexterity challenge like the tiny-pill problem?

People with Parkinson's represent a fraction of the people whose needs are unmet by mainstream health care. A huge demand for better products and services is dammed up in patient groups. Look to Seekers for a new list of priorities.

SEEKERS NEED VISIBILITY

Let's add a vertical line to our visualization of who is being served by the current health-care system, right down the middle, dividing those whose needs are *not* being met on the left and those whose needs *are* being met on the right.

At the top of the vertical axis are issues that are visible to mainstream health care. That is, people who control access to valuable resources in the current health-care system both recognize the problem and see it as their job to help. Note that there are many people who can unlock sources of power to help solve problems. Clinicians, payers, policymakers, regulators, journalists, pharmaceutical and device company executives, investors, researchers, and patients themselves each play a role.

At the bottom of that vertical line are those that are invisible to mainstream health care. Some health conditions or physical challenges appear to be unsolvable mysteries—or, to an outsider, too minor to address. People may be living in "you look fine" purgatory, without outward symptoms, clear biomarkers, or test results to prove a diagnosis. Onlookers have little or nothing to offer besides sympathy. In the worst-case scenarios, people suffering from certain symptoms and challenges are unseen and ignored completely, even by friends and family.

This is the Rebel Health Matrix (figure 3.1). It is a way to understand the full picture of suffering and the potential for improvement in the health-care system. It will also help people identify markets ripe for attention and investment.

The club that everyone wants to join is the upper-right quadrant, where people's needs are met and they are visible to the mainstream health-care system. But that club is more exclusive than it should be.

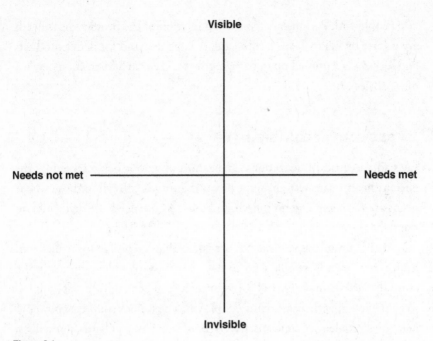

Figure 3.1
Rebel Health Matrix.

When I shared an early version of this model online, I received great suggestions about how to refine and improve it. Lisa Suennen, a health-care entrepreneur and investor, suggested that we divide the lower-left quadrant into three parts to better explain why mainstream health-care leaders are not serving some people's needs:

- because they truly do not know what to do;
- because they do not make enough money doing it; and
- because they choose not to acknowledge the problem at all.

There is overlap among these groups, but it is still useful to name them. The patient-led revolution aims to help people move up and to the right of this model, helping to spread awareness of problems that deserve attention and new pathways to well-being. Seekers are the people demanding to be heard, asking for what they need, and not giving up until their issues are acknowledged.

Wendy Lynch, a data scientist and translator, pointed out that there are three levels of visibility. The first level is to be visible to yourself. You recognize that you have a problem that is not being addressed. The next level is to be visible to people who matter to you and, in an ideal scenario, to be believed by these friends and family members. The third level is to be visible to people who can help, such as clinicians, researchers, and social workers.

Needs also have three levels. To understand your own needs is the baseline. To learn what is available and how to ask for it is level two. To get your needs met is level three.

SEEKERS NEED ACCESS TO INFORMATION

Before the internet broke open the floodgates, health information trickled down to patients, filtered by their clinicians. The best resources were kept locked up and out of reach.

One morning in 1994, the year Netscape released the first commercial web browser, the Englewood Hospital library in Englewood, New Jersey, received a phone call.[3] The caller identified himself as Dr. Harold Blakely, a local family practitioner. He gave the librarian a bibliographic citation for an article in a medical journal and asked her to make him a copy and to leave it on the table outside the library door, where he could pick it up on his evening rounds. This request was not unusual. The hospital librarians frequently left copies of journal articles that local doctors could pick up after the library had closed.

Later that afternoon, the caller phoned again, checking to be sure that his article was ready. But the library's director, Kathy Lindner, took the call this time. Lindner knew Blakely, but she did not recognize the caller's voice. After a brief discussion with a colleague, she phoned Blakely's office. After several minutes, the bewildered doctor came to the phone. He assured Lindner that neither he nor anyone in his office had called the hospital library that day.

Half an hour after the library closed that evening, a nervous, well-dressed man with carefully barbered gray hair entered the hospital through a side entrance. Walking with a cane, he passed the elevator, climbed the stairs with some difficulty, and continued down the second-floor hallway toward the medical library. As he picked up the envelope with Dr. Blakely's name on it, a hospital security guard stepped out of the doorway where he had been waiting and asked him to identify himself.

Under the questioning of the hospital's security service, he admitted that he was Edwin Murphy, a fifty-eight-year-old insurance agent with a chronic hip problem. Blakely, his physician, had been urging him to undergo a promising new surgical procedure. Murphy was intrigued but not convinced. He wanted to know more about the potential risks and benefits of the proposed procedure and had repeatedly asked Blakely to help him obtain a copy of the definitive review article, which had recently appeared in a major medical journal. Blakely had not done so. Finally, in desperation, Murphy had decided that there was only one way to obtain this vital medical information: he would have to impersonate his own physician.

Edwin Murphy was a Seeker, hunting and gathering to survive.

Paywalls still block access to the full-text versions of many journals. Motivated patients and caregivers find ways around them—emailing the article's author to ask for a copy, sharing PDFs with each other, or using a rogue website like Sci-Hub, which provides public access to millions of research papers.

In the wake of the destruction caused by COVID-19, researchers at the Johns Hopkins Center for Health Security point to "an urgent national security and public health need to ensure effective management of public health misinformation and disinformation by increasing accessibility of correct information and reducing the reach of false information."[4]

Think of all the Seekers wandering in the information desert, wishing they could find answers to their questions or a path toward better health. Their predicament is particularly galling since US taxpayers fund the National Institutes of Health (NIH), which in turn funds much of the research being kept out of their reach. Open access to research findings and high-quality information should be a priority for everyone who wants to see improvement in health outcomes.

SEEKERS NEED PLACES TO EXCHANGE IDEAS

My blog post featuring Seekers' hacks for handling tiny pills is an example of a pop-up peer group, a place where Seekers can find each other and exchange ideas without joining a formal community. Once you start looking for these pop-up peer groups you will see them everywhere. For example, Amazon reviews.

In 1995, one year after Murphy's library misadventure, Amazon.com began to allow people to post reviews of their purchases directly on the product page where other shoppers could see them. Experts and professionals were no longer the sole arbiters of quality as regular people flooded in by the millions to share their opinions.

One of the top-selling items in Amazon's Health and Personal Care section is a 7-day pill organizer with over 35,000 reviews and 80+ answered questions. People who purchased this inexpensive item came back to share their experience with what looks, to the untrained eye, like a minor purchase. The passion and detail of the reviews reveal the truth. Pill organizers can be both immensely helpful and incredibly frustrating:

"I bought 2 of these for my 95 year old father. . . . He has a tremor, his finger dexterity isn't good and his eyesight is poor but he says he finds the Ezy Dose trays easy to use. I prepare one for the week and another for the week ahead."—J. Butler, United Kingdom, reviewed January 15, 2019.

Negative reviews can be just as helpful:

"Every week I've had to pick medicine off the ground or my bag as carefully as possible because we have a toddler and this thing is not secure. Who it'd be good for: People who keep their medicine in one place. Who it would not be good for: People who have to have their medicine available on the go."—April, United States, reviewed March 17, 2021.

Health advice is being exchanged on a massive scale in Amazon reviews. Here are the bestselling items in a sample of health-related product categories and the number of reviews each one has received:

1. Mobility and Daily Living Aids: pillbox (49,000), reading glasses (76,000), seat cushion (89,000).
2. Baby and Child Health Care: gas relief drops (13,000), vitamin gummies (43,000), forehead thermometer (157,000).
3. Health Monitors: blood pressure monitor (40,000), bathroom scale (129,000), fingertip pulse oximeter (209,000).

Amazon's leaders likely did not intend for it to become a platform for peer health advice, but the sheer volume of reviews shows their customers' strong motivation for sharing what they know for the benefit of fellow patients, survivors, and caregivers.

Health-care leaders and product designers can benefit, too, if they tune into Seekers' feedback loops. Comments and reviews are an abundant, renewable resource for people looking for ways to eliminate pain points or provide better service. And they raise the public profile of common, but currently invisible, problems. If you offer health-care services or products of any kind, find ways to collect feedback directly from your customers. Learn from Seekers by listening to their questions, compliments, and complaints.

These pop-up microcommunities are wildly useful in the moment and serve as a warm-up act for more established peer health communities, when someone is ready to dig deeper. Thanks to Amazon and other online review sites, people now expect to be able to learn from peers and get just-in-time advice. And, as the next set of stories illustrates, one person speaking up about their experience can trigger a cascade of change.

Buckle up. The ride is about to get bumpy.

SEEKERS NEED SOLVERS AND CHAMPIONS

Josie King was just eighteen months old when she died from medical errors in Baltimore in 2001. Her mother, Sorrel King, channeled her grief into an advocacy campaign for patient safety. Josie's story brought tears to the eyes of anyone who heard it, but that was not enough for her mother. Sorrel King did not want her daughter's life and death to inspire emotion. She demanded that it inspire action. She went out on the hunt for ways to prevent medical errors.

Don Berwick, MD, was, in 2004, the CEO of the Institute for Healthcare Improvement. He decided to challenge clinicians in the US health-care system to prevent one hundred thousand unnecessary deaths from medical errors. And he asked Sorrel King to be onstage when he announced the campaign.

At the event, Berwick listed the changes that would be necessary to achieve their goal, including more uniform treatment for heart attacks, infection prevention protocols, and better methods for ensuring the right amount of the right drug was being given to the right person at the right time. And one more thing: a rapid response team to quickly evaluate and treat patients who are getting sicker. In Berwick's vision, it would be triggered by a nurse or other clinician.

When the microphone was passed to King, she asked, "Do you think a patient or family member could push the button? Could they call the rapid response team to the bedside if no one was listening to them and they were scared out of their minds?" The audience began to applaud, some of them rising to give King a standing ovation. She went on, saying, "I believe with all of my heart that if I had been able to call a rapid response team, my daughter Josie would not have died. She would be six years old, and I wouldn't be standing here today." She handed the microphone to Berwick, to sudden and complete silence.[5]

One team of nurses heard King speak that day and decided to create Condition H (for Help), a hotline that families of hospitalized patients can call to activate a rapid response team. Piloted at the University of Pittsburgh Medical Center (UPMC), Condition H was implemented across all eighteen hospitals in the UPMC system by the end of 2007 and began rolling out nationwide.

In the rebel health lexicon, Berwick was a Champion who recognized the brilliance of a Seeker's idea and, by sharing the scarce resource of clinicians' attention, gave King the visibility she needed to attract Solvers to her cause. The UPMC team members are both Solvers and Champions, using their skill sets and resources to build and integrate a patient-led safety initiative into their clinical practice.

The Condition H program is modeled on other rapid response teams, such as Condition A (for cardiac or respiratory arrest) and Condition C (for crisis). Clinicians on those teams run from wherever they are in a hospital to a patient's bedside to exert their authority over the situation as specialized experts, saving lives by acting quickly. Only hospital staff can activate Conditions A and C. Condition H, by contrast, places that authority with a patient's family, acknowledging that they know the patient best and may observe a downward spiral before a nurse or doctor notices.

But that power shift is incredibly awkward. Family caregivers often want to please their loved one's clinicians, whom they hold in great regard, so they stay quiet. Even doctors find it difficult to speak up on behalf of a family member, as the next story illustrates.

FAILURE TO RESCUE

While being treated with chemotherapy for a recurrence of cancer, Margaret Welch developed a severe, systemic infection. It is a well-known and highly treatable condition if clinicians act quickly.

Her son, Jonathan Welch, MD, arrived at his mother's hospital in Wisconsin to find that the window of opportunity was closing. But he didn't want to offend her clinicians. He was too polite, too reticent, and, sitting by her bedside, he watched the time slip away. His mother died a preventable death.

In December 2012, he shared his family's story in the journal *Health Affairs* as a way to extract meaning from the tragedy.[6] In the article, Welch highlighted Condition H, which was not available in the hospital where his mother was treated. He wrote about how even he, a doctor, hesitated to create a fuss, but he may have had the courage to trigger the family lifeline.

My overwhelming reaction to Welch's essay was despair. "Failure to rescue," as preventable hospital deaths are called, is devastatingly widespread. I shared a link to his article on Twitter, asking, If a clinician can't get safe care for his mother, what hope do the rest of us have?

Within days, that hope took hold in Alabama.

SEEKERS NEED COURAGE

Kyra Hagan, a health-care marketing executive, was tending to her hospitalized mother in Birmingham, Alabama. Because of an incorrect diagnosis, her mother's physicians stopped her heart failure medications. Instead, she was receiving large quantities of intravenous fluids, which, for heart failure patients, can dangerously back up into the body's tissues. In this case, Hagan's mother gained over thirty pounds of fluid in just four days. Her mother was slowly drowning as water accumulated in her lungs.

Hagan pleaded with her mother's clinicians to change course. But the health-care providers' reactions were sluggish and feeble. With each passing hour, her mother, overwhelmed by fluid, swelled like a balloon. Now unresponsive, her mother was dying in front of Hagan's eyes.

Hagan was desperate. In true Seeker fashion, she refused to believe that there was nothing to be done. She went out on the hunt. And, since she is a Networker who has honed her skills for curating community and pooling knowledge in her professional life, she began scrolling through her Twitter feed on her smartphone. There, she saw my tweet. She clicked through to read Dr. Welch's article, including his reference to Condition H. "Condition H?" she puzzled. "That sounds familiar." Looking up from her phone, she spotted a Condition H sign hanging on her mother's bathroom door.

Hagan recalls thinking, "Would this really work? What would happen if I called it and no one came, but instead told the nurse on the floor that I had called? Would I alienate anyone who might be able to help us? Should I call? How long would it take to get anything done? It's almost 4:30 in the afternoon. Would it be the next day before anything happened and could Mom survive this way for that long?"

Remembering Dr. Welch's words about different endings playing out in his mind, Hagan picked up the phone and dialed the number. The person who answered the phone was friendly and efficient. The call took less than a minute.

A few minutes later, a rapid response team rushed into her mother's room. The group quickly obtained important tests and ordered critical medications, stabilizing her mother's condition. A team member turned to Hagan and said, "Thank you for calling us. Know that you saved your mom's life today."

Jonathan Welch and Kyra Hagan didn't know each other, but he became, at that moment, a source of peer health advice. He was able to lend her the courage to pick up the phone and trigger the lifeline he wished he'd had—and that Josie King inspired. In this way, Welch is a Champion, using his powers as a clinician and writer to shine a spotlight on a patient-led solution that Hagan (a Seeker-Networker) could implement. He helped Hagan climb out of the lower-left quadrant, where her needs were unmet and unseen, to the upper right, where she got the help she needed (figure 3.2).

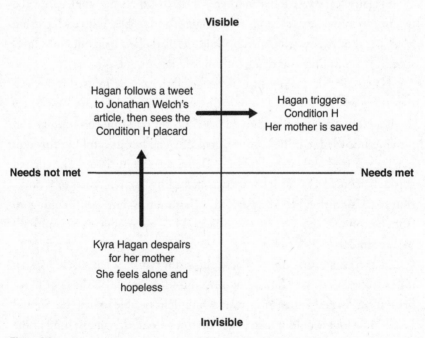

Figure 3.2
Rebel Health Matrix: Condition H.

Every caregiver desperately wants their loved one to live. One got her wish, thanks to the bravery and vision of Seekers, Solvers, and Champions who seized opportunities to act. Condition H has now been implemented by over two hundred health-care organizations nationwide.

SEEKERS NEED TO SHARE THEIR STORIES

If a Seeker has lived through a health challenge and come out on the other side with useful insights and experiences, we need to give them a way to share their stories.

Think about the stories you could tell—or amplify—that would help someone see the danger ahead in their own lives. Think about how you can provide a forum for Seekers' stories and help spur people to take courageous action or share their tips for everyday challenges, like medication management.

Connection can happen anytime, anywhere, between people whose lives intersect for a moment online, asynchronously. And that connection can have real-life consequences.

Takeaways:

1. Seekers need access to information and to each other.
2. Online reviews are free market research provided by Seekers on the hunt for what works—and what doesn't.
3. Seekers, Networkers, Solvers, and Champions can work together on life-saving solutions.

---

4 NETWORKERS

Vicki McCarrell had always dreamed of becoming a mother. When she gave birth at age thirty-eight to her son Sean, life seemed complete. Yes, he had the full facial paralysis typical of Moebius syndrome, but otherwise, he looked perfect to her. Indeed, at the hospital near her home in Van Nuys, California, she was given a diagnosis and not much else. Nobody told her how to feed a baby who could not suck or even warned her that it would be an issue.

With her husband back at work as the manager of a construction company, McCarrell was alone at home with a hungry, crying baby. She grew frantic. Sean was not getting anything down his throat no matter what she tried. She reached a breaking point when a pediatrician scolded her that Sean was losing weight as if she was not desperately worried about that exact thing. None of her friends with typical children had advice. The doctors were no help. What was she going to do?

That's when McCarrell's scrappy Missouri farm-girl spirit came out. If something isn't working right, she thought, you fix it with what you have on hand.

She went to her sewing basket, picked out the biggest needle she had—the one for darning socks—and heated it in the flame of her gas stove. She stuck it through the rubber nipple, widened the hole, and offered the bottle to her baby. Sean drank and drank.

McCarrell decided then and there to change things for Moebius families. They shouldn't have to live like castaways on a desert island, isolated and making do with scarce resources as their babies starved. She would stand in the breach between what health care can provide and what community could build. But how to begin? One neurologist told McCarrell that she would likely never meet anyone else with Moebius syndrome. It was just too rare.

But she was a Seeker. And Seekers go out on the hunt.

It was 1991, long before the widespread use of email, so McCarrell inserted a clean sheet of paper into her electric typewriter and tapped out a letter to the National Organization for Rare Disorders. She explained her situation and asked if they knew of other people with Moebius syndrome. No, they replied in a neatly typed letter but suggested writing to the National Foundation for Facial Reconstruction in New York. Within a week of mailing that second letter, McCarrell received a reply with contact information for three people, including a mother of a two-year-old with Moebius who lived just four miles away in Reseda, another suburb of Los Angeles.

More than thirty years later, McCarrell vividly remembers watching that child, Chelsey, running around and eating potato chips like any other kid. She felt hopeful for the first time about Sean's future. Together with Chelsey's mom, Lori Thomas, McCarrell started the Moebius Syndrome Foundation—the group that Nell Minow stumbled upon when she was searching online a few years later on behalf of her Uncle Burt.

McCarrell and Thomas decided not only to fix what was broken in their own health-care experiences but also to send out a beacon to guide others to their safe harbor. And with that, they stepped into their roles as Networkers.

In the early days, they scrounged for resources and built their network one person at a time. It wasn't until Thomas's daughter's "smile surgery" was featured in *People* magazine that the floodgates opened and people with Moebius all over the world were able to find their way, online and offline, to the peer community they never knew existed.

Don't assume, though, that the internet era has solved this problem. Anyone with a mysterious set of symptoms can tell you that they feel as isolated and alone as McCarrell did in 1991. The difference now is the speed with which people can form a group and get the word out *if* they find each other.

This chapter is about how Networkers build infrastructure for the patient-led revolution, whether they face a systemic failure or a personal earthquake. The path has been broken and the foundation has been laid for a more responsive health-care system. It is up to us to expand on these pioneers' work.

NETWORKERS GATHER AND SHARE INFORMATION

Thanks to the internet, people are now able to gather information and collaborate anytime, nearly anywhere, with everyone who has something to contribute. Here's a story about how the doors swung wide:

In 1968, Stewart Brand began publishing the *Whole Earth Catalog*, a quirky collection of product reviews and ordering information for things like food grinders and camping equipment. The first issue was thin, just thirty-one pages, but grew every year as Brand added listings for every kind of useful tool he and his editors could find.

The *Whole Earth Catalog* was a way to disseminate specialized information, connect far-flung communities, and empower people to try new things. It was like an early paper-and-ink prototype of the internet.

In the mid-1980s, Brand and others seized the opportunity to create an online trading post for ideas, called the Whole Earth 'Lectronic Link, or WELL for short. Usenet and other early online communities were created around the same time, precursors to commercial platforms like America Online. People could communicate, in real time or asynchronously, at any time of the day or night.

Howard Rheingold, an early member of the WELL, wrote,

> In a virtual community we can go directly to the place where our favorite subjects are being discussed, then get acquainted with people who share our passions or who use words in a way we find attractive. In this sense, the topic is the address: you can't simply pick up a phone and ask to be connected with someone who wants to talk about Islamic art or California wine, or someone with a three-year-old daughter or a forty-year-old Hudson; you can, however, join a computer conference on any of those topics, then open a public or

private correspondence with the previously unknown people you find there. Your chances of making friends are magnified by orders of magnitude over the old methods of finding a peer group."[1]

True to its roots in San Francisco's counterculture movement, one of the biggest communities on the WELL was devoted to the Grateful Dead, a band that traveled with its own tie-dyed tent city of fans and followers.

Connection became a commodity to be created and traded as people discovered that uncanny feeling of being understood by someone you may never meet face-to-face. Everyone could share what they know and learn from one another.

In 1989, public radio producer Jay Allison wrote an essay about caring for his fragile, sick baby daughter and finding the parenting group on the WELL: "At 3:00am my 'real' friends were asleep, so I turned to this foreign invisible community for support. The WELL was always awake. Any difficulty is harder to bear in isolation. There is nothing to measure against, lean against. In typing out my journal entries into the computer and over the phone lines, I found fellowship and comfort in this unlikely medium."[2]

The parenting group weathered the illnesses of other members' children, collectively hunting and gathering information, sharing their experiences, and borrowing expertise when they needed it. In this way, they were harkening back to their great-great-grandparents' practices of families supporting each other through hard times, knowing that when they needed help, the community would rally around them too. As Networkers, they were spinning those practices forward in ways their ancestors could not have imagined.

UNCHARTED TERRITORY

In the early days of the online health revolution, the internet frightened a lot of clinicians, as people started gathering, sharing, and creating information with each other—unsupervised. It was as if patients were piling onto ships bound for the horizon, and clinicians were holding maps showing that the world was flat. Medical authorities saw people sailing toward the limits of knowledge, and they honestly thought patients might fall off the edge into an abyss of misunderstanding.

One group of researchers decided to gather data.

In May 2001—the first year that a majority of American households had internet access—the *Journal of the American Medical Association* published a landmark study measuring the accessibility, quality, and reading grade level of health information found online. Researchers gathered information using the same method a consumer might: by typing simple phrases into a general search engine.

They found that less than a quarter of the first page's search results linked to relevant material. Much of it did not meet clinical guidelines for accuracy, particularly if the search was conducted in Spanish. And it was written at such a high reading level, many Americans would not be able to easily understand it.[3]

Their findings were alarming, but the worst was yet to come from a clinical expert's perspective. Regular people—untrained armchair health experts—started writing on blogs, in online discussion groups, and other patient-led outlets. People were using the internet to share intimate and specific personal health experiences. This seemed inherently dangerous to some clinicians, and in December 2001, the American Medical Association released a statement suggesting that Americans make a new year's resolution to "trust your physician, not a chat room." But people continued to flock online, gathering, sharing, and creating health information.

Unfortunately, misinformation does thrive online. Scoundrels post unfounded claims and lead people astray. The unwary fall into traps laid by anti-science activists. But when the stakes are high, it is possible for people to band together and raise their game. They form far-flung study groups, pooling their knowledge and keeping each other as up-to-date as possible on the latest research. That's the essence of the story of how the tide started to turn toward greater respect for community-led information resources.

NETWORKERS CROWDSOURCE THE TRUTH

In 2005, *Nature*, a respected journal, conducted a peer review of a broad array of scientific articles published by *Encyclopedia Britannica* and Wikipedia—and found that they were essentially equal in accuracy.[4] A high-quality information resource could indeed be created without professional editorial oversight, and "disputes about content are usually resolved by discussion among users."

Health researchers decided to test a hypothesis put forward by patient advocates who claimed that a healthy online community weeds out bad information, and that discussion forums can be a source of high-quality health information.

A team of clinicians analyzed the content of an online breast cancer forum and found that 10 of 4,600 postings were false. But forum participants corrected seven of the misleading posts, often within a few hours.[5] Only three posts containing misinformation went unchecked by the community.

The addendum includes excerpts of the ten "bad" postings. They show that this was a high-level medical discussion among people whose lives were at stake. Group members talk about prescription-drug shelf life, disease-staging parameters, and the likelihood of recurrence within five years—serious topics, taken seriously. The excerpts show that patients, when given access to sound medical information, cite it and put it to use.

This finding matches the study I shared in chapter 1 showing the value of peer advice related to ICD treatment. Among the hundreds of conversations, researchers found eighty-two examples of participants giving each other medical advice, most of which was benign or helpful. In a separate study of members of an online community of people with diabetes, nearly 40 percent said they had been helped by following advice found in the group, and 99 percent reported no harm.[6]

Online health communities are an information market opportunity, not something to disparage or dismiss. The desire to seek advice and collaborate on solutions is an unstoppable force. We need to channel it, not try to dam it up. We need to give people tools to defend themselves against misinformation on a personal level. And technology companies need to do a better job of removing accounts that spread falsehoods at scale.

Those early pioneers of online health communities were building the infrastructure for an unthinkable challenge: a pandemic.

LONG COVID

Fiona Lowenstein became sick from the COVID-19 virus in March 2020. Their symptoms lingered and did not follow the path described in news accounts. As the founder of Body Politic, a queer, feminist health collective, Lowenstein was already part of an online peer community. They created a special subgroup to track an emerging phenomenon: Long COVID.

Lowenstein shared their story in the *New York Times*, urging young people to take the virus seriously. It garnered nearly one thousand reader comments. Then, in a follow-up piece published in the *Times* one month later, Lowenstein detailed long-term symptoms that were not yet being recognized by the World Health Organization (WHO) and other public health officials: fatigue, headaches, congestion, sore throat, short-term memory loss, and other challenges. As they wrote, "When I first came home from the hospital, I felt alone in my healing process. I wanted information, and to connect with others who shared my experience, so I started an online support group for people experiencing COVID-19 symptoms or recovering from the virus."

Lowenstein threw a pebble into the public conversation about COVID-19, and a tidal wave of pain and affirmation came back.

People all over the world responded to these and other first-person testimonies, joining Body Politic, Survivor Corps, and other online peer communities. More "long-haulers" shared detailed records of their symptoms online. More news outlets began covering the phenomenon, widening the circle of awareness. Long COVID patients connected their struggle with existing post-viral illness groups, such as people living with myalgic encephalomyelitis/chronic fatigue syndrome (ME/CFS). Together, these communities gained strength and clout, garnering the attention of the WHO, the US Centers for Disease Control and Prevention (CDC), and NIH. A new radical health movement rolled toward mainstream recognition, sparked in large part by media coverage of what *patients* were doing, beyond what establishment medicine had noticed.

Alone, people with Long COVID slipped through the cracks. Together, they formed a net to catch each other. They built the missing infrastructure.

Peer connection can feel like finding someone who speaks your language in a foreign country. It can be deeply satisfying and even cathartic to find someone else who has had the same troubles, frustrations, and small victories. To know you are not alone is powerful. You might be better off, or you might be worse off by comparison, but either way, you will benefit from the people who have traveled the path before you.

Peer health communities help people find not only possible treatments but also answers to questions like, "Given my—or my loved one's—limitations, how can we build a happy life?" Experienced Networkers can fill in knowledge gaps and act as a backstop against misinformation or miscalculation. They can help someone new to a chronic condition begin to manage it on their own.[7] Remember Natalie Abbott's praise for the Moebius community: "Hope comes through connections, resources, strength, and time, instead of in a pill. But hope is as valuable as a cure." Hope pulls you toward communities of peers who can start to answer your questions and meet some of your needs.

Experienced Moebius parents show new ones how to feed their babies with facial paralysis, helping some of them to avoid the complications and expense of surgically placed feeding tubes. And, since many people with Moebius live with low dexterity and limb difference, Networkers gather and share tips like how to stick a pen through a tennis ball to make it easier to grip. They pull themselves and others out of the lower-left quadrant of the Rebel Health Matrix (needs not met, invisible) over to the lower-right quadrant—but in these cases, their needs are met thanks to fellow Networkers, not mainstream health care.

By contrast, people living with Long COVID started in the lower-left quadrant (needs not met, invisible) and, thanks to their own research, documentation, and organization, they've pulled themselves up into the upper-left quadrant. They still have unanswered questions and unmet needs, but at least researchers and clinicians are beginning to acknowledge the validity of their experiences. Lowenstein leveraged their talents as a writer to gain visibility for their fellow Seeker-Networkers. By doing so, they attracted both Solvers and Champions to join their alliance (figure 4.1).

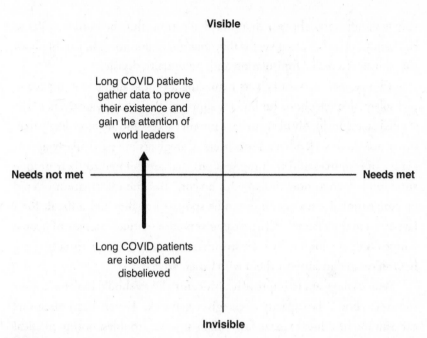

Visible

Long COVID patients
gather data to prove
their existence and
gain the attention of
world leaders

Needs not met ——————————————————— Needs met

Long COVID patients
are isolated and
disbelieved

Invisible

Figure 4.1
Rebel Health Matrix: Long COVID.

NETWORKERS HELP PREVENT COMPLICATIONS

Imagine that you have not slept in days. You can't remember when you last ate more than a handful of pretzels or a protein shake from the nurse's station. Something terrible has happened. But your loved one is alive. Now it is up to you to decide if they get to come home or if they will live out their days in an institution. Not able to abide the alternative, you choose to bring them home. You are given a rudimentary introduction to a sophisticated piece of medical equipment and then you are left alone, at home, with no further instructions. The night stretches ahead, and you listen to the ventilator, breathing for your loved one. Will you ever sleep through the night again?

Thanks to medical and technological advances, more patients are now able to leave the intensive-care unit and go home with a mechanical ventilator or "vent."[8] It's better for everyone—except the caregivers. The vent user gets to be home with their family, and payers reap the savings since home care is significantly cheaper than hospitalization. But the burden shifts to the family and other caregivers as they maintain, monitor, and troubleshoot the vent. It is a recipe for isolation and, potentially, disaster.

Twenty years ago, caregivers managing a vent at home would have to rely solely on a telephone hotline for support. These days, caregivers in the United States are highly likely to have internet access and are more likely than other people to seek advice from peers. Caregivers are particularly appreciative of resources and training sessions that are tailored to their unique situation—such as how to live with a vent.[9] But the information offered by conventional sources online can be spotty in quality and difficult for a layperson to understand.[10] These caregivers are a sentinel example of people whose needs are not met by mainstream health care. The peer-to-peer safety net can catch and support them with expert advice.

People who want to improve health-care delivery should look for opportunities to boost the capacity of caregiver networks. Experienced caregivers can run the health-care maze faster than anyone, troubleshooting medical equipment problems, managing medications, and preventing mishaps. They are an untapped resource *and* a group that is hungry to find ways to keep their loved ones safe.

NETWORKERS INCREASE VISIBILITY FOR THEIR ISSUES

Imagine a magnet at the top of the Rebel Health Matrix pulling people off the horizontal line depending on whether their problem is visible to the mainstream health-care system or not. For example, people whose needs are not being met might be pulled into the upper-left quadrant because the health-care system at least recognizes their predicament. Networkers may have gathered evidence and amplified their voices to raise the profile of their community. Clinicians and scientists may even have ideas about how to solve the issues the community faces. Still, good news may not have spread to everyone who needs to hear it. Again, Networkers can help increase visibility of both problems and solutions. They can build the magnet that pulls themselves and people like them up into the top half of the grid.

The club that everyone wants to join is the one in the upper-right quadrant where people's needs are met and the health-care system both sees them and knows how to help. Questions are answered. Cures are at hand or solutions are straightforward, like a broken arm that can be set and stabilized. The /r/STD subreddit is an example of how Networkers can help pull people out of the lower-left quadrant (no clue about what to do, not yet connected with the health care system) up into the upper-right quadrant by giving science-backed advice ("that's a treatable infection, go see a clinician right away"). We need to build more platforms and give people more tools to safely give and receive high-quality peer health advice (figure 4.2).

Imagine a magnet pulling downward, to the world where mainstream health care is not much help. The most dismal prospects are among those who find themselves deep in the lower-left quadrant: their needs are not

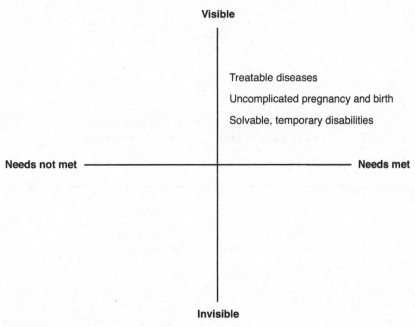

Figure 4.2
Rebel Health Matrix: Visible, needs met.

being met and they are essentially invisible. They may not yet even recognize that they have a problem—the deepest level of obscurity.

NETWORKERS POOL RESOURCES

If people whose needs are not being met can find each other, they can rally together and become Networkers. In this way, they can start to at least answer each other's questions and slowly migrate up or to the right side of the chart, where their problems are more visible to mainstream health care or some of their needs are being met (figure 4.3).

For example, when device companies denied Dana Lewis's request for a louder CGM alarm, she was stuck—at least for a while—in that lower-left quadrant. Then, thanks to networking and know-how, she built a custom solution and pulled both herself and her community over into the lower-right quadrant. By publishing a book, journal articles, and countless tweets

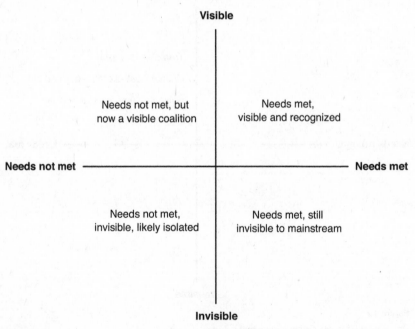

Figure 4.3
Rebel Health Matrix: Four categories of visibility and need.

about her work, Lewis increased the visibility of the diabetes rebel alliance, which drew more people to the cause. Together, they pulled themselves up toward mainstream recognition.

A MASSIVE MARKET

People whose needs are not being met by the current health-care system are aching to get their questions answered or simply be recognized as having a problem worth solving. This is a massive market encompassing millions of people (figure 4.4).

Again, in this model, only the people experiencing pain, discomfort, or confusion get to decide if their needs have been met. They alone judge if their questions have been answered. This is one way that people take back power: by refusing to accept an answer or a treatment until they are satisfied.

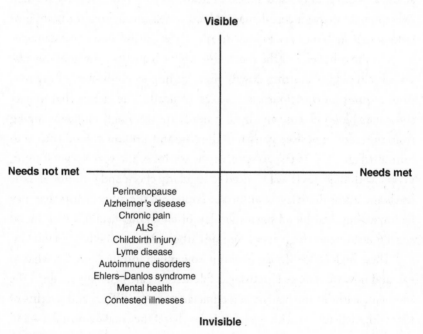

Figure 4.4
Rebel Health Matrix: A fraction of the health concerns crowding the bottom-left quadrant.

For example, to an outsider, diabetes appears to be a solved problem in health care. There are well-known drugs, therapies, and practices that work. But people who live with diabetes are mad as hell about the clunky systems they live with, and some of them are not going to take it anymore. Refusing to accept the status quo, they band together to innovate their way out of it.

But first, a quick primer.

A HIGH-STAKES, CONFUSING SLOG

Diabetes is a life-limiting condition characterized by the body's inability to produce or use insulin, a hormone that enables glucose to be used by the body's cells for energy. Over thirty-four million Americans live with diabetes, including 5–10 percent who require regular doses of insulin to stay alive.

Insulin needs change frequently—sometimes from day-to-day or even hour-to-hour. If your blood sugar is extremely high, your blood becomes acidic and can lead to acute illness or death. If your blood sugar stays high over time, the extra glucose damages blood vessels throughout the body, ultimately causing blindness, kidney disease, heart disease, and nerve damage.

On the other end of the spectrum, if your blood glucose goes too low, your brain begins shutting down, often leading to confusion, disorientation, seizures, unconsciousness, strokes, or death. The factors that impact someone's blood glucose and insulin needs are seemingly endless, ranging from the amount of sleep you get to the type and amount of food you eat to hormonal changes, stress, exercise, or the season of the year. To get it right, people with diabetes (PWDs) need to regularly check and monitor glucose levels and assess those levels within the context of the other factors that may be impacting their blood sugar that day, often taking insulin if their blood sugar is heading too high or consuming carbohydrates if it is headed too low.

These high-stakes decisions about how much insulin to inject, what to eat, and how to manage blood sugar fluctuations are generally made in the moment, without the benefit of a clinician's advice. PWDs and parents of kids with diabetes live with the knowledge that if they make a mistake—and don't catch it in time—there could be dire consequences. And the pace never slackens. They worry about blood sugar levels twenty-four hours a day, seven days a week. They have to read ingredients, measure portions, and calculate if the carbohydrates they eat are "covered" by the medications they take. Living with insulin-requiring diabetes is a frightening, confusing slog.

Community-based groups led by trained peers, like those organized by the YMCA, have been shown to be effective in helping people prevent and manage diabetes. There is also a vibrant online community of people living with diabetes. Those who tap into it benefit greatly from the camaraderie and the information exchanged.

Anna McCollister, an entrepreneur who lives with insulin-requiring diabetes, says, "The best way to get the knowledge you need to keep your blood sugar steady and stay healthy is through other patients. Before the internet, doing that was very difficult. If you were lucky, you might meet one other person with diabetes, but that person likely had a very different body and life than you. Finding somebody who was truly like you was nearly impossible—until the internet."

If human connection could be bottled and sold, it would fly off the shelves. We need to make it easier to find. We need to build the missing infrastructure of well-being.

PATIENTS START SHOWING UP

When Amy Tenderich was diagnosed with Type 1 diabetes in 2003, she was a freelance journalist and mother of three living in California. She looked

---

Tip for Aspiring Networkers: Listen First

You may feel hesitant about joining a community. Maybe you've sworn off Facebook, Twitter, and other social platforms. That's OK. Podcasts are a great way to dip into a topic and start to pick up terminology, as are YouTube videos. Listening and learning from others like you can make you feel like you are part of a larger community.

Search YouTube and your favorite podcast service for the same key words you are using to consult Dr. Google. Subscribe to one or two podcasts or video channels. Expand the list when you are ready.

---

online but found very little useful, actionable information. Undaunted, she launched DiabetesMine in 2005, a blog that captured her questions and answers—and thousands of readers and fans. She created the resource that she wished she had as a Seeker and then set about creating an ecosystem of innovation, powered by people living with diabetes.

At the time, most companies and organizations were not aware of bloggers' growing influence, especially among people who are otherwise unconnected to each other, like PWDs. Tenderich's negative review of one ham-handed marketing campaign by a major pharmaceutical firm dominated that company's search results for two years—to the dismay of executives who did not even know who she was.

As she recalls, "For many years, medical device companies considered their customers to be clinicians. They would go to clinicians to ask if a new product had clinical value but they never ran it by the people who had to live with it, who would have to wear it 24 hours a day." The same was true for national organizations like the American Diabetes Association. People at the top of the power structure did not see the patients coming. But come they did, showing up online and in person at events.

Networkers organized themselves into communities on social platforms. Some focused on liberating device data. Others raised questions about the cost of diabetes supplies and insulin. Everyone contributed to the diverse, supportive pageant of life inside the diabetes online community (DOC). They identified and increased the visibility of problems that were not yet being solved by mainstream health care and, by doing so, pulled themselves into the upper-left quadrant. Patients and caregivers built the infrastructure for diabetes care that our health-care system otherwise lacks (figure 4.5).

PEERS HELP. A LOT.

Networkers can save health systems money and accelerate improvement. But recommending peer support still feels new and risky to health professionals who have not had time to read all the studies that might assuage their fears and convince them to recommend that their patients connect with a community or peer coach.

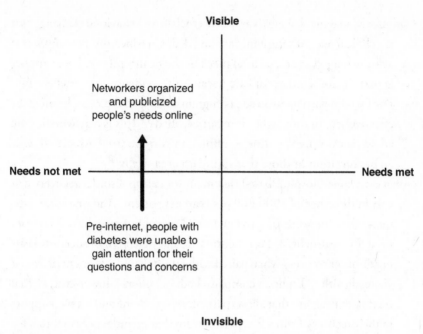

Visible

Networkers organized
and publicized
people's needs online

Needs not met ———————————————————————— Needs met

Pre-internet, people with
diabetes were unable to
gain attention for their
questions and concerns

Invisible

Figure 4.5
Rebel Health Matrix: Diabetes.

There is a rich, deep evidence base, spanning at least forty years, that shows the benefits of connection among patients and caregivers. A sampling:

Arthritis: Participation in an arthritis peer group yielded benefits that lasted for years, including a mean decline in reported pain of 20 percent from each patient's baseline and 40 percent fewer clinical visits. A comparison group, not part of the peer-led self-management program, did not report the same benefits.[11]

Complex chronic conditions: Weight loss, smoking cessation, and other behavior changes require sustained effort. Most people cannot break or form new habits alone. Peers for Progress, a public health program affiliated with the University of North Carolina, reviewed the literature and found that social, emotional, and daily management support from a community health worker or other trained nonprofessional can help people successfully navigate a range of complex conditions, from cardiovascular disease to drug, alcohol, or tobacco addiction.[12]

Diabetes: Managing diabetes is as much a social and behavioral challenge as it is a clinical one. Among clinicians and diabetes educators, peer support is acknowledged as an essential piece of the health puzzle. Peer support is part of the standard of care because the evidence is overwhelming: PWDs who participate in such programs managed their condition more effectively than those who were not enrolled.[13] This is true whether the advice is exchanged online or offline, in communities associated with an organization or those that spring up organically.[14]

Eating disorders: Hospital-based treatment for eating disorder recovery can cost in the range of $900,000 per year, per patient. And one study estimates that "between 67 percent and 83 percent of cases have an unmet need for treatment."[15] Peer mentors are a key element of successful eating disorder recovery when paired with family-based treatment delivered via telehealth.[16] Equip, a company I advise, offers a lower-cost, virtual treatment program that allows patients to stay home and receive support in their recovery from a five-person team that includes peer mentors for both the patient and their family members.

Mental health: The strong evidence in favor of peer support led the Centers for Medicare and Medicaid Services to recognize it as an effective intervention for mental health.[17] Peer counseling is also endorsed by the American Psychiatric Association and the Veterans Health Administration. For example, people cycling in and out of psychiatric wards have been paired with trained "recovery mentors" who themselves had experienced major mental illness. During a nine-month study, people assigned a peer mentor had fewer hospital admissions and spent less time in the hospital than those who received usual care (i.e., no peer support).[18]

Organ transplant: Organ recipients and their caregivers were invited to join a private Facebook group set up by clinicians at the University of Cincinnati where they spent nine months asking questions, getting advice, and sharing information about recovering from transplant surgery. Nearly everyone (95 percent of survey respondents) reported that joining the group had a positive impact on their care, and 97 percent reported that their main motivation for joining was to provide or receive support from other patients.[19]

Pregnancy: Social support is an essential ingredient to a healthy pregnancy, particularly if the support comes from other experienced parents and people who have recently given birth, whether their counsel is provided online or offline. Fifteen of seventeen studies looking at peer support in maternal and child health recorded a significant, positive effect when compared with people who received no such support. Good social support is even predictive of fetal growth and a baby's birth weight.

This sample demonstrates the wide range of health conditions that benefit from firsthand, community support. There is always room for further research, but there is enough evidence to merit investment and action.

Takeaways:

1. Social support can be as nourishing as tactical advice. Peer health communities organized by Networkers provide both.
2. Peer connection can yield measurable health benefits, especially among people with chronic conditions like arthritis, diabetes, and mental illnesses.
3. People whose needs are not being met can rally and become a more visible coalition, more likely to be recognized—and served—by mainstream health care.

---

5 VISIBILITY AND COMMUNITY

Dave deBronkart held a piece of paper in his hand. Life as he knew it was collapsing around him as he absorbed his kidney cancer diagnosis. And his doctor was inviting him to go online.

It was 2007, and Dr. Danny Sands was among the few clinicians in the world prescribing peer health communities like the Association of Cancer Online Resources (ACOR), a collection of email-based conversations or LISTSERVs. ACOR had been started in 1995 by Gilles Frydman after his then-wife, Monica, was diagnosed with breast cancer, and the best information they found was online but disorganized. By 2007, ACOR encompassed 160 groups and 55,000 members worldwide.

That one recommendation to connect with other people living with kidney cancer triggered an avalanche of goodness for deBronkart. The community welcomed him, made him realize he was not alone, answered his initial questions, and recommended that he get in touch with one of the four clinicians in the greater Boston area who were using the only treatment available in those days that had a small chance of saving him: HDIL-2. As it happened, he was already seeing one of the four.

DeBronkart later found out that most kidney cancer patients had never heard of this life-saving protocol because the leading database for treatment options, the National Comprehensive Cancer Network, contained information that was years out of date. One oncologist told deBronkart that his research showed a 7 percent response rate and a 4 percent death rate from HDIL-2. The ACOR community, however, knew that the most recent data demonstrated a 25 percent response and just 1.5 percent mortality. The hospital where deBronkart received treatment had an even better ratio of survival: they had a 30 percent response rate and had lost just one patient in the last 1,200 treated. Online, experienced kidney cancer patients and caregivers showered deBronkart with advice about how to prepare for and recover from the tests and treatments he faced. He credits his doctor's "ACOR prescription" as one of the turning points in his life.

Online communities of patients and caregivers are crucial to the success of the patient-led revolution. We need the door to be as wide and welcoming as possible, drawing in everyone who can benefit or contribute.

This chapter outlines how to help people link up with others like themselves and become Networkers. The sooner they do, the sooner they can get better care and—if they choose—contribute to the revolution.

NETWORKERS NEED TO TALK TO STRANGERS

Some people have never met a stranger. They are able to chat with anyone, anywhere, and learn something. Others are less likely to strike up a conversation with people they don't know. They underestimate the value of what they could learn. Or they underestimate people's interest in helping them. Aspiring Networkers need to know that both of these barriers are false.

Research shows that if people expect to learn something useful in conversations with strangers, they are more likely to do so. By contrast, people with low expectations are less likely to try—and they, therefore, miss out on everyday learning opportunities.[1] Those who hold skeptical views about talking with strangers ought to overcome their hesitation. You never know who may be holding the tidbit of information, connection to a clinician, or "been there" advice that you need.

The other false barrier that holds people back is their hesitation to ask for help. Research shows that people overestimate the burden they place on others when they express a need and underestimate the benefits that accrue to helpers, who feel good about themselves if they pitch in.[2] Practice asking for help in small ways so that you will be ready when the time comes to network your way to the care you need.

Some people may feel alone because they do not fit a typical image of a person living with a chronic illness. Or their disability is not visible. They are hidden in plain sight.

Liz Salmi, who was diagnosed with a malignant brain tumor in 2008 at age twenty-nine, wrote about the challenge of finding a community of peers:[3]

> About four weeks after my first brain surgery I decided to go to my first cancer support group meeting. I thought it would be a good idea to meet other people like me . . .
>
> I imagined we'd trade notes and complain about healthy people with day jobs. This was not the experience I had.
>
> I sat in a circle with a social worker and about 10–15 people old enough to be my mom. The group's participants represented a diverse cross section of the cancer community: Various cancer types, retired folks, people with kids and grandkids, those still working, people in treatment, people done with treatment. Some were "cured" but were still scarred by their cancer experience and came for moral support.
>
> "Hi, my name is Liz, and I have brain cancer."
>
> I moved from face-to-face, looking for a sign of recognition, looking for someone who knew what I was talking about, but all I got were weird stares and sad expressions.
>
> Women had tears in their eyes and men shook their heads.
>
> "But you are so young," they said. "What a shame."
>
> "Seizures? Why do you have seizures?" they asked.
>
> I realized I never wanted to go to a general cancer support group again.
>
> On the way out I asked the social worker if there were any brain cancer groups. She handed me a list of about 200 groups around the greater Sacramento region. Just one group focused on brain tumors.
>
> I needed to head to the internet to find all of you.

In February 2012, Salmi helped start the #btsm (Brain Tumor Social Media) hashtag on Twitter, taking inspiration from the #bcsm (Breast Cancer Social Media) community established in July 2011.

Disease-specific hashtags on social platforms are like lighthouses guiding boats to a safe harbor. They give structure to an otherwise chaotic online conversation, helping Networkers connect with each other. The hashtag communities also give clinicians and researchers a chance to listen and contribute in a public forum. A survey of the #bcsm community found that patients who participate in discussions report an increase in understanding of their condition and a decrease in anxiety.[4]

But, of course, you need to be a user of that social platform and know what communities to look for—yet more barriers to those who want to connect with peers. This is an opportunity for anyone interested in improving health outcomes to promote useful online communities and hashtags. Networkers are out there, hoping to find a port in a storm. Shine a light.

NETWORKERS NEED SKILLFUL LEADERS

Early on in the life of an online community, natural leaders and hosts emerge. They may be a tiny minority of users but are the most likely to reply to posts, to boost the confidence of newcomers and infrequent visitors, and to guide the discussion toward topics that are appropriate for patients and caregivers (as opposed to questions best addressed by clinicians). They are what's known as "superusers,"[5] and, as researcher Anna De Simoni put it, "Ten superusers can sustain a community of 1,000 users."

Colleen Young, online community director of Mayo Clinic Connect, has noticed that members who share their most private worries and vulnerabilities can also help knit an online community together. The more people disclose, the more likely the group coalesces around a shared mission and the more likely the community will grow and last.

Her observations resonate with a pattern documented by researchers studying group dynamics: the first ten minutes of their first meeting can affect a group's problem-solving ability for the duration of their time together.[6] A meeting that starts with stiff formality breeds rigid hierarchies and roles, which is not conducive to nimble, creative work. Self-disclosure, on the other hand, builds psychological safety. It allows people to share what they know and be open to others' input.

NETWORKERS NEED SUPPORT

Mayo Clinic Connect recognizes the importance of its superusers and invites them to become part of the "Connect Mentors" program. These volunteers are often happy to give back to the community, without any expectation of pay or other reward. They help others the way they themselves have been helped and become part of the infrastructure supporting the patient-led revolution.

But even the most enthusiastic people can burn out. If we are serious about building and nurturing peer health communities—and I argue that we must get serious—we should invest in supporting those who lead them.

The #bcsm (Breast Cancer Social Media) community on Twitter is an example of the dangers of relying on unpaid volunteers. One of the cofounders died in 2016 and, ten years into this "labor of love," the other cofounder became "a constant point of contact for those with questions and concerns, well outside the bounds of the weekly chat times."[7] The two remaining moderators struggled to come up with ways to engage a broad-based population of thousands of patients. Not surprisingly, participation in the community—measured by the number of tweets using the hashtag—dipped in recent years. This is, unfortunately, a common pattern in peer health communities. The last official #bcsm chat was held on July 11, 2022.

Here are six ideas from community members and leaders about how to support the work of building infrastructure for the patient-led revolution:

1. Provide a place for community moderators to discuss common challenges, like how to handle unsolicited marketing pitches and "trolls" (troublemakers who want to disrupt the conversation).
2. Set boundaries around the volunteers' time. Nobody should feel like they have to be on call 24/7.
3. Remind volunteers to add their peer health community work to their professional résumés.
4. If moderators are paid, disclose that fact and the funding sources.
5. Allow moderators to set their own schedules, including no minimum requirement for hours.
6. Talk about succession planning. If a leader should need to step down, who is trained and ready to take their place?

Tip for Networkers: Become a Better Fact-Checker

A team of clinicians, patient advocates, and other experts in the United Kingdom developed a tool to help people judge a publication's reliability. The DISCERN instrument consists of fifteen questions that anyone can use when looking for advice about treatment choices. In evaluating a publication, a reader should ask questions like, "Are the aims clear?" "Is it clear when the information used or reported in the publication was produced?" "Does it refer to areas of uncertainty?" (It's a good sign if the authors admit they don't know everything.)

The Medical Library Association recommends starting a search at a reputable site like MedlinePlus or Healthfinder, both of which are maintained by the US government. If you can't find what you need, contact a medical librarian.

When you do see bogus advice being shared, debunk it. Tim Caulfield, a professor of health law and science policy at the University of Alberta, argues that it is worth making the effort to correct misinformation. He recommends leading with facts and making your point in a clear, authentic, shareable way so it can spread further than the one conversation you are in at that moment.

The peer health innovation ecosystem suffers every time we lose a community. We must support the moderators and volunteers who keep them up and running.

NETWORKERS NEED EASY WAYS TO FIND EACH OTHER

Facebook is a default choice for many health-related groups because it is so easy to start and build a community. Plus, if you want to catch fish, you fish where the fish are. Nearly three billion people are monthly active users and four hundred million people worldwide are part of a Facebook group they find meaningful.

The platform is specifically designed to attract people and keep them online, feeding the network with photos, videos, and status updates.

Facebook groups and private forums can feel cozy and safe. But there are downsides: outsiders don't know the groups exist and will never benefit from the insights shared. Many groups are private—not closed to advertisers, nor from Facebook's surveillance apparatus, but from the people who might benefit since neither a Facebook search nor a general internet search will expose it to a newcomer.

There are also often multiple Facebook groups focused on the same disease or condition, but because they remain separate and disconnected they never pool their knowledge. And the rebel health ecosystem misses out on newcomers' contributions because they never find the door to these private clubs.

NETWORKERS NEED DR. GOOGLE TO HELP

Just like smart urban and campus planners pave the paths that people are already walking on, we should look at where people go when they need answers to health questions. These days, it's Dr. Google.

Nearly everyone in the United States (93 percent according to surveys) has access to the internet. Of those, about seven in ten have looked online for health information, including the specific advice they can get from people who share the same conditions and concerns. One-third of US teens and young adults say they have connected with health peers online and, of those, 91 percent said it was helpful to do so.

Liz Salmi, the brain cancer survivor, points out that because more people with health questions are finding each other on social platforms, particularly in Facebook groups, the number of patients and caregivers sharing about their experiences on the open web, such as on a blog, has decreased. Nowadays, if someone searches the web for "what is it like to have brain surgery," they are more likely to find Salmi's blog post from 2008 than any first-person testimony from a recent patient who may have benefited from a new technique or treatment but has only posted about it in a private group.

Salmi says, "The shift to short-form posts increases the ease by which people can provide peer health advice, but that advice is not as easy to find for the newbies. How do we get the new patients to start blogging? Should we? Surely there are newer voices people should be listening to and learning from."

Helping people to become Seekers and Networkers is a two-sided market challenge. Leaders across the spectrum, from patient advocates to healthcare executives, need to not only build demand and encourage people to ask questions but also find ways to increase the supply of robust peer health communities.

There is not currently a trusted guide to help people judge the quality and usefulness of the information and support being shared online. Networkers and Champions can step into this breach and boost the signal for the patient-led online communities they know, but a more powerful solution would be for search engines to find ways to guide people.

NETWORKERS NEED ALTERNATIVES

Facebook currently dominates the online health community landscape. But patient-led groups exist on every social platform, from YouTube, Instagram, and Twitter to Reddit and TikTok. Podcasts, articles, and books are another way for people to learn that they are not alone in their diagnosis or health challenge, especially if there is a community popping up around the original media. A vibrant comment or review section can be a window into a previously hidden alliance of like-minded people.

How to find them? Look for hashtags and keywords. People gather around a health hashtag like it's a campfire, ready to share stories or seek advice. Some patients' social media posts inspire hundreds and even thousands of reactions and comments from people all over the world. Champions with access to mainstream media resources and other influential channels should find and amplify the most useful communities.

NETWORKERS NEED CUSTOM-BUILT PLATFORMS

Specialty online platforms like Health Union, The Mighty, Savvy Cooperative, PatientsLikeMe, and Smart Patients were built to pool patients' knowledge and data. Of the thousands of health communities that exist, some empower patients who want to help discover and refine new treatments. Others simply create space for connection and conversation.

Name recognition helps. Patients and caregivers often trust well-known groups, such as the American Lung Association or the Arthritis Foundation. Those are two of the 110 organizations that use the company Inspire as their peer-to-peer community platform. With 2.2 million members, half of whom are active on a monthly basis, Inspire is a stocked fishing pond for people looking for insights on a wide range of questions. Patients and caregivers can search across communities for tips related to, for example, surgery recovery. Researchers—both patient-led and clinician-led—use platforms like Inspire to recruit hard-to-find participants for clinical trials.

Mayo Clinic Connect is another example of a health community with enviable name recognition. Initially founded in 2011 as a marketing tool for world-famous clinical centers, one early measure of its success was the number of clinic appointments made by online community members.

In 2016, the Connect team shifted its strategy to emphasize collaboration, and there are now over one hundred thousand members from across the world. Professional moderators work with volunteer mentors to keep discussions safe, supportive, inclusive, and useful. Mayo Clinic now recognizes the peer communities as an extension of its mission to make the world a healthier place and to contribute to the advancement of science. The communities benefit from the halo effect of the Mayo Clinic's name recognition and brand identity.

Peer health groups, whether they are commercial or nonprofit, using an existing or a custom-built platform, represent a growing market. But it has not reached its peak. There is room for new entrants, particularly ones that can build platforms for collaboration, where people can track and share data, conduct a survey, or work together on a document.

Six in ten US adults live with at least one chronic condition, and most are not yet part of a peer patient community. That is 125 million people in the United States alone. This is a massive, untapped market for connection.

NETWORKERS NEED CLINICIANS' HELP

It was a golden moment when Dr. Sands handed Dave deBronkart that piece of paper—his "ACOR prescription."

Many people feel like they don't have the need—or permission—to look online for peer health advice. They say they trust clinicians. They want to believe that doctors have all the answers or worry that seeking a second opinion online will offend their primary clinical team. This is why it is essential for clinicians and other health-care leaders to recognize the value of peer health networks and recommend them to patients and caregivers.

But not everyone is going to be as savvy and connected as Sands, a Champion of peer support and patient-led innovation. Clinicians are already overworked and do not have time to find and evaluate patient-led

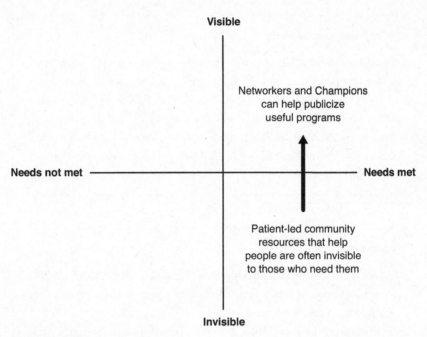

Figure 5.1
Rebel Health Matrix: Online communities.

communities and other resources. In response to this need, the United Kingdom's National Health Service pairs primary care doctors with "link workers" who know what services and support groups are available in their communities.[8] In Colombia, the Keralty Foundation works with "community connecters" to identify resources such as, for example, a salsa-dancing club in the park to get someone on their feet and exercising again. We need to expand the scope and impact of all community health programs to include peer-to-peer support and advice (figure 5.1).

People are in need. They are looking for ways to navigate the health-care maze, and most will search online at some point in their journey, stumbling into a pop-up peer group or an established patient-led community. For many people, an opportunity to connect with others like themselves is all they have wanted and all that they think they need. But then someone in the group has an idea they want to share, a way to make life better. That person is a Solver.

Tip for Champions: Stock Up

Clinicians and other Champions who want to promote peer support need to have access to a wide array of community groups that are ready to receive new patients. As public health expert Lisa McNally points out, "Just as a doctor's prescription can only improve health if the patient has access to a well-stocked pharmacy, so social prescribing schemes depend on a well-stocked community." If you have influence, find peer health communities that you can confidently recommend.

Takeaways:

1. Millions of people are already part of patient-led communities, whether on Facebook or health-focused platforms. But there is still room for growth and improvement.
2. Networkers burn out if they are not supported—a risk that can be mitigated with investment.
3. Clinician recommendations can accelerate adoption of peer support.

6 SOLVERS: TREATMENT INNOVATION

In 2008, Francesco Fornai, a researcher at the University of Pisa, published results from a study showing that lithium slowed the progression of paralysis among sixteen people living with amyotrophic lateral sclerosis (ALS).[1] The international community of ALS researchers, clinicians, and patients was riveted. There are so few bulwarks against this disease that slowly robs people of the ability to move, talk, eat, and, eventually, breathe. Many people living with ALS are willing to try almost anything, particularly as paralysis sets in.

Facing death, a Brazilian man named Humberto Macedo took a desperate chance. He asked his doctor to help him experiment with the off-label use of lithium and, at the same time, began to gather a group of fellow self-experimenters online, using the website PatientsLikeMe (PLM) to share their results.

On PLM, people maintain a profile that tracks both treatments and observations of daily living such as diet, exercise, sleep, and mental state. It's a bit like a dating service profile crossed with a clinical trial, and participants are grouped by disease.

When the lithium trial began, the dating analogy came to life: each of the patients taking lithium was paired with other ALS members according to stage of disease, calculated by their ability to talk, salivate, swallow, use utensils, walk, breathe on their own, and other key measures.

It was a complicated process, based on a complete history of each patient's illness. Those who abstained from taking lithium would constitute the "control" for their matched partners in the experimental group. Everyone agreed to track motor function and, poignantly, instruct a family member to notify PLM in the event that they died.

Months passed as 447 ALS patients, 149 of whom were taking lithium, carefully tracked the progression of their disease. In the restrained tone required by scientific publication, Paul Wicks, then PLM's director of research and development, and his coauthors described the outcome of their innovative community science project, finding "no effect of lithium on disease progression." However, they pointed out, their study "reached the same conclusion as subsequent randomized trials, suggesting that data reported by patients over the internet may be useful for accelerating clinical discovery and evaluating the effectiveness of drugs already in use."[2]

In other words, the treatment did not work, but the platform did.

Patients taking lithium reported the same level of motor function as patients who were not taking the drug. But they had their answer faster than most scientists could complete the recruitment phase of a standard clinical trial. And for patients who face a median survival of two to five years from the onset of symptoms, time is of the essence. PLM showed that those with the most at stake—patients themselves—can contribute to the science that could save their lives.

This chapter is about how Seekers, Networkers, and Solvers form teams and pursue solutions, fueled by hope. They establish patient-led working groups to find answers to questions that keep them up at night—or that threaten their very existence. Learn from these pioneers about how to spot opportunities to improve care.

Patients are traditionally seen as passive sources of data, not active participants in the research. As a result, we miss out on promising avenues of inquiry. It is time to widen our lens to include patient-led research.

PANDEMIC INNOVATION

The COVID-19 pandemic is an example of how a crisis can put a spotlight on and accelerate patient-led innovation. People infected with the virus and those caring for them were dropped into a strange new world with no map and no compass. But there were glimmers of light as Seekers and Networkers stumbled forward, virtually calling out to each other, often on social media platforms.

Patients began to find each other and start trading stories. Networkers gathered strength and expertise in community, whether their focus was prevention, treatment, recovery, or sometimes just empathy.

Solvers emerged. They scoped the problems. They brainstormed solutions. They began to build tools, like symptom trackers. Importantly, they set their own priorities and defined their own taxonomies of what *they* found important, what *they and their peers* felt was worth tracking.

Solvers and Networkers used online platforms to share innovative solutions for home care and infection control, like air purifiers made from a box fan and filters available at hardware stores. New peer-to-peer resources for disseminating scientific information were created, such as patient-led You-Tube channels, Twitter feeds, Facebook groups, and websites.

Members of Body Politic's support group for Long COVID patients saw that no mainstream authorities were tracking this emerging illness, characterized by symptoms that lingered for weeks and months, so they decided to do it themselves. They formed a small team—the Patient-Led Research Collaborative—and kept costs low by using free online tools like Slack, Google Docs, Twitter, and Facebook. They combined the expertise of Seekers, Networkers, and Solvers within their ranks, leveraging the strengths of each type of patient rebel to go out on the hunt, pool resources, and attack problems. They designed an online survey, recruited 640 respondents, collected data, and published the first research report on prolonged COVID-19 symptoms.

Because they paid attention to the questions being asked by patients themselves, the Patient-Led Research Collaborative uncovered novel observations:

- Nearly half of people reporting symptoms of Long COVID had never been tested for the virus. One in four tested negative despite reporting symptoms that matched those who tested positive. The difference was in the timing of the test: the earlier it was conducted in their illness, the more likely they tested positive.

- Symptoms fluctuated and were not limited to the widely recognized fever and cough. Long COVID patients reported neurological, cardio-vascular, and gastrointestinal issues. Since testing was limited at first to those reporting respiratory distress, medical authorities were excluding large portions of the infected population from the official count; anyone with other symptoms was being ignored by the establishment.

Emboldened by their success, the Patient-Led Research Collaborative designed and fielded a second survey, more in-depth than the first. Respondents were offered documentation of their answers, which they could take to doctor's appointments—a useful record since their official medical charts often contained very little detail about the trajectory and flavor of their illness. Other patient-led groups concerned with the long-term effects of COVID-19 formed on Facebook and other social platforms.

People with Long COVID rebelled against their status as isolated, passive patients. The Solvers among them used everyday tools to gather clinical-strength data. By doing so, patients made Long COVID a recognized condition.

NEEDS NOT MET

Long COVID patients, like so many other Seekers, were disbelieved and disrespected because their symptoms were mysterious and no name existed yet for what ailed them.

Long COVID's trajectory from obscurity to widespread acknowledgment set a new speed record in peer health innovation. Within weeks of finding each other and forming a research collaborative, their findings were sought after by medical professionals around the world.

In the Rebel Health Matrix, they started in the lower-left quadrant. Then, thanks to the efforts of Networkers and Solvers in the Long COVID patient groups, they moved into the upper-left quadrant, where their needs are still not being met, but they are at least visible to mainstream health care (figure 6.1).

Long COVID patients still lacked support of nearly every kind: financial, political, legal, and social. But they were starting to be believed.

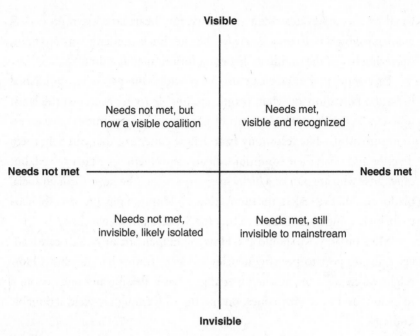

Visible

Needs not met, but
now a visible coalition

Needs met,
visible and recognized

Needs not met ———————————————— **Needs met**

Needs not met,
invisible, likely isolated

Needs met, still
invisible to mainstream

Invisible

Figure 6.1
Rebel Health Matrix: Four categories of visibility and need.

A NEW PARADIGM

Belief in the truth of a patient's lived experience is a leap that doesn't always get made in health care. Symptoms go unreported on a chart because clinicians are under tremendous time pressure or because they simply misunderstand. Clinicians are trained to listen and yet still can't always hear what someone is trying to say, much less capture it in the medical record. Plus, being new to illness or unused to fatigue can make it hard for a patient to know what to pay attention to or how to explain it. That's why it is important for people who are suffering to learn how to find each other, online or offline, and gain the observation and tracking skills they need to effectively describe what is happening. Being in community sharpens the senses, helping people recognize and report common patterns.

For example, even people with well-known health conditions report symptoms that do not fit the stereotype. About 40 percent of women having a heart attack do not experience chest pain, but it is the first warning sign listed on most websites when you search for "heart attack symptoms." A woman having a heart attack may feel like her bra is suddenly way too tight, squeezing her in the middle of her chest for minutes at a time.

Peer-generated advice can also help bridge the gap when published literature falls short or when people are unable to get access to the latest updates. Networkers who are part of peer health communities have access to information—like testimony from fellow patients—that can help them describe and track their conditions. Again, a problem might get solved, but only those who are part of a lucky in-group will get the news through social platforms. That's a leak in the innovation-to-adoption pipeline that we need to fix by helping more people to become Seekers and Networkers.

More broadly, we should ask, How might mainstream health-care leaders tune into peer-to-peer frequencies and learn from what they hear? How might we create a new research paradigm that is flexible and open enough to include everyone with a question and rigorous enough to yield actionable findings?

To put it bluntly, we have been looking for our keys under the streetlamp because that's where the light is shining. We need to widen the lens of biomedical research and get creative, particularly in a fast-moving, unpredictable situation like a pandemic or in the drama of a personal earthquake like a life-changing diagnosis.

A RIGHT TO TRY TO SAVE YOUR OWN LIFE

There is precedent for patient-led biomedical research. The rebel alliance ACT UP illustrates how people with little or no training can pull themselves up out of the invisibility of the lower-left quadrant (needs not met, no seats at the research table) and then over to the upper-right quadrant (highly visible, able to influence both policy and clinical research). Let's frame the story using the four archetypes of the patient-led revolution:

Seekers: In the early 1980s, people began to fall ill from a mysterious new disease. They had nowhere to turn for answers. Clinicians, scientists, policymakers, and community leaders were confused and disorganized in their responses. Seekers from within the community most deeply affected by the illness went out on the hunt.

Networkers: Gay men and lesbians were among the first groups to create grassroots organizations to address the epidemic. They gathered and shared information about prevention, testing, and treatment as quickly as it could be validated. Networkers pooled resources.

Solvers: Peer-led groups began organizing politically and demanding attention for their questions and concerns. Community-based patient and physician partnerships created new pathways for treatment discovery and knowledge-making that were faster than the traditional, government-funded process. Solvers attacked problems.

Champions: AIDS activists established themselves as credible experts on biomedical research and drug policy. Champions inside the federal government took up their cause and began to fast-track innovations.

Steven Epstein captured the drama in his book, *Impure Science: AIDS, Activism, and the Politics of Knowledge*.[3] In 1987, patient-led research groups, frustrated by the slow pace of government action, asked Anthony Fauci, MD, then the director of the National Institute of Allergy and Infectious Diseases, to change federal guidelines to recommend a promising drug (pentamidine) that early studies showed was effective in preventing a serious fungal infection (*Pneumocystis* pneumonia or PCP). He said no, citing a lack of data, so the activists set out to test it on their own. Two years later, the US Food and Drug Administration (FDA) approved the treatment, based solely on community-based research—a milestone for the patient-led revolution (figure 6.2).

Around the same time, ACT UP emerged as a powerful, peer-led organization. Chapters were typically independent of each other and operated by consensus, with no formal leaders. They demanded changes at the federal level, particularly at the FDA, which controlled access to experimental drugs. Peer-led organizations also innovated grassroots importation and distribution hubs to get "drugs into bodies."

Dr. Fauci, who was initially hesitant, evolved in his thinking and urged fellow researchers to partner with patient-activists, saying, "When it comes

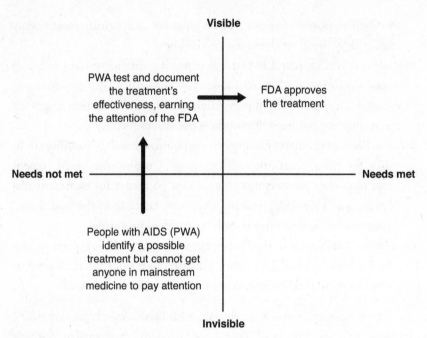

Visible

PWA test and document the treatment's effectiveness, earning the attention of the FDA

FDA approves the treatment

Needs not met ———————————————— Needs met

People with AIDS (PWA) identify a possible treatment but cannot get anyone in mainstream medicine to pay attention

Invisible

Figure 6.2
Rebel Health Matrix: HIV/AIDS in the 1980s.

to clinical trials, some of them are better informed than many scientists can imagine."[4] He benefited from the work of his deputy, James Hill, who was gay, HIV-positive, and acted as an ambassador between patient-led activists and government officials.[5] The rebels brought outsider perspectives to insider discussions and contributed to the science that would save people's lives.

SELF-TRACKING

Long COVID and HIV are examples of emerging conditions that were so new that they had not yet been defined, much less measured, before they tore through the population. Patients themselves collected and analyzed data to prove their conditions' existence and to demand research funding.

Other times, the mystery is a private matter. An individual decides to document symptoms and map the terrain of their health, whether they plan to explore it alone or with the help of clinicians. People also gather data about themselves in order to make positive changes, like increasing their stamina or improving the quality of their sleep.

Self-tracking is a low-cost, effective intervention. A study I led in 2012 found that 7 in 10 US adults are tracking some aspect of health, their own or someone else's.[6] Most people are interested in tracking weight, diet, or an exercise routine—the basics of well-being. A smaller group tracked higher-level health indicators or symptoms, like blood pressure, blood sugar, headaches, or sleep patterns. Half of the trackers keep notes on a regular basis and the other half wait until something crops up, like a symptom flare or a new goal. Many said they do not keep detailed notes (instead of tracking their exact weight, for example, they just try to fit into their favorite jeans). One-third of trackers used pencil and paper, like a notebook or journal.

More recently, researchers at Rock Health and Stanford University's Center for Digital Health found that 83 percent of adults in the United States track some aspect of their own health. Most (65 percent) use a digital log or journal, a wearable, or a connected medical device.[7]

In the realm of clinical advancement, researchers demonstrated that patients tracking their own symptoms during cancer treatment both live longer and feel better, possibly because clinicians are able to respond more quickly to problems identified by close attention to changes.[8]

PERSONAL SCIENCE

But even with the greater availability and sophistication of tracking devices and tools, this instrumentation still falls short when it comes to solving some health mysteries. People are not always sure where to begin or what to measure.

One answer to this challenge comes from the Quantified Self community, a network of individuals who formulate their own research questions, design studies, collect observations, and look for patterns. They are Seekers, Networkers, and Solvers engaging in self-tracking and measurement, a practice that has come to be known as "personal science."[9]

Rather than focusing on the population-level aspects of health research, personal science is an individual pursuit. Practitioners share methods and ways of seeing, and, as Quantified Self founder Gary Wolf writes, "each person's success makes the next success easier."[10] This is one of the strengths of the patient-led revolution, whether it is people tinkering with medical devices or solving their own health mysteries. Personal scientists pursue their own goals and share what they learn. Again, these rebels are prosocial, not anti-science.

For example, Sara Riggare, PhD, lives with PD and that sometimes means handling tiny pills at the exact moment that she is most likely to be clumsy—when she needs her medications. Based on the data she collected using personal science methods, she saw that taking her pills on a strict schedule helps control her symptoms. She devised a highly individualized exercise and care plan that includes a stackable pill organizer she can fit in her purse so she can reduce the number of late or missed pills.

Riggare, a Seeker and Networker as well as a Solver, is constantly on the lookout for new techniques and treatments. One day, in a Facebook group, she saw a video posted by Jasmine Sturr, who successfully experimented with nicotine as a way to control the involuntary muscle movements called dyskinesia that are associated with PD. Sturr had read a study in which researchers induced PD symptoms in squirrel monkeys and then reduced the animals' dyskinesia by dosing them with nicotine. Trained as a chemist, she replicated the protocol for herself at home.

Together, the two personal scientists, Riggare and Sturr, devised a placebo-controlled, single-subject experiment to see if nicotine would have a similar positive effect on Riggare. Indeed, it did, lifting her brain fog and reducing her dyskinesia.

CREATIVE SOLUTIONS

Riggare continually experiments and shares her findings. For example, she has publicly documented her successful use of a walking stick and a rollator walker to prevent falls. She has also published her self-tracking findings related to COVID-19, physical activity, and dexterity challenges. She has not written up some of her more offbeat, but just as useful, interventions, such as wearing a knee pad only on her right knee. The pad makes her less fearful of falling and thus makes her more confident, which has a direct effect on her ability to stay upright. She has also found that jumping on a trampoline reduces the number of times she "freezes" (a well-known PD symptom). Riggare is a Solver who adapts all kinds of gear to serve her purposes.

People living with disability and their care partners are constantly adapting home health equipment to meet their needs. These personal scientists tweak and experiment, inventing, customizing, and—if they are Networkers as well as Solvers—sharing their innovations with others. Applying ingenuity to physical challenges and then sharing those home health hacks is an activity worthy of mainstream attention and resources. By improving their own mobility, making a home safer, and creatively solving everyday problems, people with disability save themselves and the health care system money.

Personal science skills are useful for identifying emerging health issues and for managing complex, ever-changing conditions. Everyone, whether living with a chronic condition or not, should learn how to begin a personal science project in case they face a question they—and mainstream health care—cannot answer.

Leaders should tune into the conversations happening among personal scientists. Their explorations of what is possible in their own health could yield actionable, system-wide insights.

Tip for Solvers and Networkers: Build Your Skills

People do not respond uniformly to illness or to treatments. You need to find what works for your body, your schedule, your budget.

Pick one aspect of your health, like a symptom or measure you care about. If you want to make a change, try one thing at a time and track the effects. Learn more and build your skills by downloading the ebook *Personal Science: Learning to Observe* by Gary Wolf.

If you are a Networker, or aspiring to be one, find fellow patients who have tried different techniques, treatments, and devices. Be ready to share your own questions and observations when an opportunity presents itself.

RISK MITIGATION

Online exploration can be dangerous, of course. Sham treatments are discussed online every day, and lives are put at risk when people are lured into those dark corners of the internet. We must give people the tools and support they need to ward off misinformation as they explore their own health questions. The more we can connect patient-led, personal science to the traditional biomedical research model, the faster we will make progress. If we do not, people will continue to test the limits of safety if they think it will help.

For example, in an online peer discussion group, Brett Alder read story after story shared by other men who share his condition, POIS. Their testimonies of brain fog and inflammation provided much-needed relief from his emotional burden: he was not alone.

After getting to know others in the group, he introduced the topic of self-treatment using subcutaneous immunotherapy, the protocol that Dutch researchers outlined.[11] Injecting a diluted amount of an allergen is an increasingly common way to treat allergies. In this case, it would be a man's own semen. Two men in the Netherlands had been successfully treated this way. Despite having no medical training and no support from his clinicians, Alder was determined to replicate the protocol at home.

Some members of his online group were encouraging. Others voiced concerns about the risks of unsupervised therapy such as anaphylactic shock, a systemic allergic reaction that can be fatal.

Several men decided to move forward, including Alder, without any professional medical oversight and no control group besides their own health history. As much as I admire their bravery, I wish they had been able to find clinicians willing to oversee the experiment.

Happily, Alder's story ends well. Encouraged by his peers, he began the protocol that relieved his symptoms. His early struggles are becoming a distant memory. Alder and his wife, Jenica, now have nine children.

DIY MEDICINE

As long as there are people whose needs are not being met by mainstream health care, there will be people like Sturr, Riggare, and Alder freelancing treatments based on their reading of the scientific literature, whether the intervention involves something relatively benign, like nicotine, or potentially hazardous, like self-injection of an allergen.

Anna Wexler, an assistant professor at the University of Pennsylvania's School of Medicine, studies the ethical, legal, and social issues around do-it-yourself (DIY) medicine and citizen science. She identifies four key factors for the rise of DIY medical movements: a population of individuals who are suffering, the ability to quickly and easily communicate with each other, lack of access to an experimental treatment, and an ability to create the therapy or build a device without special equipment or materials.[12]

Wexler notes that skepticism among clinicians and professional medical societies is a significant barrier to citizen science gaining traction in some quarters. As she writes, "Even physicians who may see the value in collecting crowdsourced data may be hesitant to get involved with DIY medical movements, either due to fears of being associated with a fringe movement or due to concerns about liability (i.e., in terms of providing medical advice to patients or assisting them with procuring supplies)." Among all the communities Wexler tracks, only one currently shows promise for breaking through to more widespread acceptance: the DIY diabetes movement.

Takeaways:

1. Biomedical research has a blind spot. People living with a condition should be seen as partners—even leaders—in investigations into the health challenges they face.
2. People living with disability and their care partners are creatively overcoming everyday physical challenges.
3. Personal science can yield fresh ideas for one's own well-being, as well as new or improved treatments and devices.

---

7 SOLVERS: DATA ACCESS

When Ben West was diagnosed with diabetes in 2003, his doctor prescribed a glucometer, a portable insulin pump, and a notebook. West dutifully called in his handwritten notes to his clinician's office each night but quickly realized that nobody was doing anything with the data. It was up to him. He set about understanding the devices that were keeping him alive.

He asked the manufacturer for the pump's documentation (a guide to code that runs it) but they said no. That's when West decided to try, with the help of his sister and father, to reverse-engineer the insulin pump, breaking it down, piece by piece, in their living room. West and his family had joined the diabetes rebel alliance.

In 2014, West showed Dana Lewis and her partner, Scott Leibrand, how to send commands to the pump to administer insulin. Lewis and Leibrand then took it a step further and figured out how to forecast and account for fluctuations, using publicly available data on insulin activity.

As Lewis writes, "Within a few months, we had evolved from a simple, 'louder alarm system' to essentially having built an algorithm and an 'open loop system' that suggested insulin dosing adjustments and carb corrections. We didn't know it at the time, but this was the precursor to the first open source closed loop algorithm that would later be known as OpenAPS."[1]

Yes, that's right. Their collaboration yielded a DIY, open-source artificial pancreas system (OpenAPS) two years before the FDA approved a similar device manufactured by Medtronic.

The diabetes hackers published what they had done online, for free, and people around the world began cobbling together their own systems to link or "loop" their devices together. Thousands of people have built their own OpenAPS rigs, sometimes using older devices because newer models have more restrictions on the data access points that the diabetes Solvers rely on.

This chapter is about what is possible when people get access to the tools and data they need to solve their own problems.

DATA TAKES CENTER STAGE IN DIABETES

A little background is in order. In 1999, the FDA approved the first CGM for consumer use. Patients insert a tiny sensor under their skin so the CGM can track glucose levels in subcutaneous tissue. The device then sends that calculation to a separate receiver. Crucially, CGMs collect data every five minutes of every day, so people can track trends in their glucose levels and respond quickly to changes. These devices are not covered by all health insurance plans, nor are they recommended to every patient.

For those able to obtain one, the CGM replaces the cumbersome process of regularly pricking their finger to test blood sugar using a handheld meter. Even better, it gives the user a steady stream of information about where their blood sugar is, where it has been, and, importantly, where it is going next and how quickly it is changing.

With traditional blood glucose tests, patients get a static picture of where they are at the moment of the test. With a CGM, patients see not only where they are but also trend lines that can be critical in helping make decisions about exercise, food choices, and insulin needs.

In addition, a patient can set alarms on their CGM to alert them if glucose is going too high, too low, or changing very quickly. CGMs provide an important measure of protection for patients with insulin-requiring diabetes, especially those who live alone, providing life-saving alarms and alerts to wake patients who may otherwise have slept through a life-threatening episode of hypoglycemia.

The first generation of CGMs were designed to keep the data locked in the hardware, which was the industry standard for all monitoring devices, whether they were keeping watch over a human's blood sugar levels or an oil refinery's process control loops. Users had to be physically in the same room with the device to see the data. These monitors were designed to honor the old and outdated model of data management: lock it down tight.

The attitude of diabetes device manufacturers was paternalistic, asking, essentially, "What would a consumer do with the data? It's safer in our hands." Their other argument was that if consumers had access to the data, then the device company's competitors could also gain access and reverse-engineer their technology. Protecting the data was a way to protect their market share.

But this cut off the possibility of user-driven innovation around the management of diabetes. It also blocked data from flowing between and among devices—what the health-care industry calls "interoperability." The people who know best what they need—PWDs and their loved ones—were not allowed to try to solve their own problems. And other innovators were not able to create platforms, apps, or other services to fill in the gaps left by the entrenched, slow-moving device companies.

A MATTER OF LIFE AND DEATH

This keep-out attitude has had serious implications. How many people suffered for years because they did not have access to the data to build their own solutions, like Lewis's louder alarm? What is the cost to society when we do not allow people access to the data, information, and tools they need to solve problems?

When I speak at conferences, I tell the story of the diabetes data liberation movement as an example of the entrepreneurial spirit that abounds in patient and caregiver groups. I share Lewis's story as a parable of the patient-led revolution and invite people to learn more about the wide network of expert patients, caregivers, and clinicians who share her mission to create solutions for people living with diabetes.

Sometimes it's hard to know how a story lands with an audience.

One day, about a week after I had shared Lewis's story in a keynote, I received an email from a woman who said she wanted to raise her hand during the Q&A, but couldn't. She wrote,

> I had a couple questions to ask you, but frankly was unable to speak as one of the patient stories you shared had me fighting back tears. A close friend from high school lost his brother at only 21 years old. He was a Type 1 diabetic with a CGM that didn't wake him to adjust his insulin when he was home sick with a cold. It was so tragic, and the excuse given was that he was overly sedated with over-the-counter cold medicine, and the manufacturer could not be held responsible as it was unusual circumstances of use. I totally understand why the #WeAreNotWaiting group exists, and I only wish it had been around 15 years ago so he would still be with us.
>
> Human stories really are what drive us, and the least we can do is honor those that have gone before us by informing and motivating ourselves to make sure we prevent this from continuing to happen as best we can.

Her story should motivate all of us to keep working toward an open-data future for health care. The hashtag she refers to—#WeAreNotWaiting—is a rallying cry specific to the diabetes community.

The phrase was coined by Lane Desborough, a diabetes dad (D-dad) who was frustrated with clunky technology, and the social media hashtag was created by another D-dad, Howard Look. Desborough, along with Ross Naylor and Kevin Lee, collaborated with John Costik to launch the Nightscout Project in 2014—an amateur diabetes surveillance system created by and for people who use CGMs.

Because of their work, blood sugar data could be sent, for example, to a parent's smartwatch so they could monitor their child's levels while at school, on a field trip, or at a friend's house. A community sprang up online, and people began teaching each other, peer-to-peer, how to set up Nightscout for themselves, which is the only way to stay on the right side of the FDA. Under US law, an individual can experiment on themselves—or their child—but not on anyone else. As one Solver puts it, "In my house, I am the FDA." PWDs pulled themselves up into the upper-right quadrant where their needs are now visible, documented, and—among those able to wrangle the devices—met (figure 7.1).

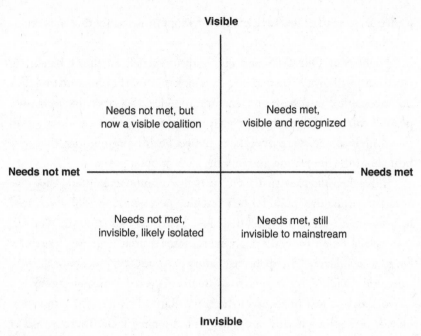

Visible

Needs not met, but
now a visible coalition

Needs met,
visible and recognized

Needs not met ———————————————————————— Needs met

Needs not met,
invisible, likely isolated

Needs met, still
invisible to mainstream

Invisible

Figure 7.1
Rebel Health Matrix: Four categories of visibility and need.

OUTSIDER INNOVATION

Sometimes, when people connect with others who share the same health challenges, entrepreneurial teams emerge and the ideas start to flow. Seekers, Solvers, and Networkers push each other to greater heights. They thrive in community with each other.

Without social platforms like Twitter and the support of the DOC, John Costik's tinkering with his son's CGM would not have spread to other patients and families. It would have been nearly impossible for his insights and know-how, honed in upstate New York, to reach Dana Lewis in Seattle. And she would never have had the chance to build her own diabetes alarm system, much less the revolutionary OpenAPS.

The internet gives us access not only to information but also to each other. It allows people to share their concerns, to find out that they are not the only ones who are exhausted and frustrated. And as people gather together, they become a visible coalition—evidence of an underserved market, ready to adapt and adopt innovations that make their lives better.

Nightscout, OpenAPS, and all the advances made by the DOC add up to a triumphant story: frustrated Seekers look online. The ones who find each other become Networkers and start trading ideas. Solvers come up with a possible solution. When they are ready, they share it, and Networkers spread the word. If someone is part of the right peer health communities, they may hear about the innovation and join the early adopter group.

This rebel alliance sees diabetes as their common enemy, and they give away everything they build for free, teaching newcomers the skills they need to make their own or their children's lives better. As Costik put it, "For me, commercialization was never an option because I'd rather help twenty or thirty families now than hold it up in a regulatory or some other process for the next three years" and then get beaten to the market by a big company anyway.

But that is just one side of the story. Radical patient-led innovation outside the existing health-care system is not for everyone. There are lots of people who do not have the technical skills or courage to build their own remote monitoring system or loop their devices together. Or their clinicians warn them off even trying because of the very real risks associated with setting it up incorrectly. Some innovators choose to follow a more traditional path, partnering with a commercial entity that can scale their inventions to hopefully benefit millions of their fellow patients and caregivers—not just the pioneers and hackers. The patient-led revolution needs both outsiders and insiders to push the industry forward.

BIGFOOT

More than a year before John Costik freed his son's CGM data to set up remote monitoring, Bryan Mazlish had done the same thing for his wife, Sarah, and son, Sam, both of whom live with insulin-requiring diabetes. But they had not shared their accomplishment on public forums as they continued to test and refine it. Mazlish also successfully rigged together an artificial pancreas system for his loved ones but again kept it secret. They knew the stakes were very high and wanted to be sure they had the system exactly right.

Rumors of these audacious feats and his commitment to anonymity led *Wired* magazine to call Mazlish the Bigfoot of diabetes hackers in 2014, after the mythical elusive monster.[2] He was not shy, though. He was early.

Mazlish had built a successful career in quantitative finance, modeling stock market data to guide trading. Like others in the diabetes community before him, he had been appalled by the locked-down, inflexible devices that his wife used to manage her condition. The Mazlishes had an ongoing, friendly debate about whether a computer could manage some aspects of diabetes better than a human can, but since Sarah was a clinician (and lived with the condition), Bryan stayed on the sidelines.

Things changed when their son Sam was diagnosed with insulin-requiring diabetes in 2011. All of a sudden, Bryan was in the game. Sarah managed Sam's blood glucose levels during the day, and Bryan took the nights. He set alarms and stumbled down the hallway every three hours so he could peer in the dark at Sam's CGM screen. "Will I ever sleep through the night again?" Mazlish thought. There had to be a better way.

A YouTube video fired his imagination. It showed a contraption that hovers a camera over a CGM, presses a button on the device, and then emails an image to a parent or care partner. It was clunky, but it would mean that Mazlish could at least stay in bed when he woke up to check Sam's levels.

Excited by the prospect of remote access, Mazlish started exploring how to incorporate optical character recognition into his plans. It would be an imperfect patch added to a barely acceptable workaround, like taking a picture of a page and then using software to translate the image back into text and data. His brother-in-law, an engineer, listened to Mazlish's plan, nodded, and asked a crucial question: "What does that jack do?"

It was the CGM's charging port and, essentially, a backdoor into the device's data storehouse. After a few days of testing, they gained direct access.

Within a year, the Mazlishes had perfected their homemade artificial pancreas rig. They sought advice from Jeffrey Brewer, then the head of the powerful diabetes advocacy group JDRF (formerly known as the Juvenile Diabetes Research Foundation), who connected them with regulators at the FDA. The FDA warned the Mazlishes that while it was fine to create solutions for their own family's use, any attempt to share their know-how—even for free—would be illegal. The CGM was classified, at the time, as a Class III medical device (meaning it is life-supporting or -sustaining) and subject to the highest level of scrutiny by the federal government.

"One genesis of my success is understanding the rules, understanding where the line is, and pushing it as far as it can go, but not breaking the rules," says Bryan, recalling their disappointment. "Once we had talked with the FDA, it was over. There was no plausible deniability."

The FDA was not ready for the patient-led revolution in 2012. And instead of asking for forgiveness, not permission, as many rebels do, the Mazlishes had sought the federal government's guidance. And the feds said no.

For the next two years, Bryan Mazlish shopped their innovation to commercial partners and was even willing to give it away for free, just to see more people benefit from it. The "Mazlish box" was used in clinical trials in the Netherlands, but no commercial device makers saw it as a priority. They could not see what Mazlish and other people living with insulin-requiring diabetes saw: an end to their nightmare of sleepless nights and gnawing worry. Their needs were not being met by mainstream health care, yet their pleas for help fell on deaf ears. They were stuck in the lower-right quadrant of the Rebel Health Matrix, where a problem has been solved for their family, but the solution was invisible—or being ignored—by people in power.

Mazlish teamed up with Brewer to start a company to build solutions for this gaping hole in the market. They named it Bigfoot Biomedical because who could resist such a moniker? One of their early collaborators was Lane Desborough, who observed that Bigfoot Biomedical took what was a mystery and made it a puzzle—and a puzzle can be solved, eventually.

Mazlish is quick to point out that he did not invent anything. He pulled together assets and information that had been developed in academia to create a DIY proof of concept. He was bending rules, not breaking them, which fit with his and his wife's experiences working inside the highly regulated industries of finance and medicine. They wanted to share their innovation widely, but they also did not want to defy the federal government. As individuals, they were stuck. As a business, the team of Solvers behind Bigfoot Biomedical could move forward.

DATA ACCESS IS ESSENTIAL

The diabetes data liberation movement is a sentinel example of what happens when people find out that someone is blocking their access to a vital resource. Individuals burrowed their way into the data trove and shared know-how with their fellow rebels; teams started building the tools they needed to live better with diabetes.

But diabetes devices are a tiny slice of the health data market. Think about all the medical devices and consumer-grade wearables collecting data on people's symptoms and activities. Think about all the medical record data that exist in hospitals, research institutions, and clinicians' offices. Think of all the devices tracking the quality of our air, water, and other environmental factors of health.

Once you start looking across the landscape of health data, you will see that our current understanding and access fall woefully short.

Picture a map of the world drawn in the fifteenth century by European cartographers. They could depict the coastline of Italy in loving detail while most of Africa and Asia remained indistinct blobs. The Americas and Australia are missing altogether. This was the best that the mapmakers could do with the data they had. Explorers kept sailing off to the edges of the world known to Europeans, coming back to share what they found, and the maps improved. That is how we need to approach health data. We need to recognize that we do not yet know what we will discover. We should not block access to people who want to explore the edges of what is possible. We must not fall into the trap of capturing what we see today and proclaiming it to be what exists.

Tip for Solvers: Stay Outraged

Lots of innovation has stemmed from someone getting angry, frustrated, or outraged about the situation they find themselves in.

Write a manifesto. What are the worst aspects of the challenge you face? What would you change first, if you could? Channel that energy toward creating a solution.

MY BODY, MY DATA

Hugo Campos was thirty-seven years old when he collapsed on a train platform in San Francisco in 2007. He recovered and, for three years, trusted his clinicians who assured him that it was a blip and not worth worrying about. This was exactly what he wanted to hear, so he believed it. Plus, as he recalls, "I was completely unprepared, so I trusted."

A second collapse forced Campos to come to his senses. His true condition, hypertrophic cardiomyopathy, is a common form of genetic heart disease that affects an estimated one in five hundred people. "Hypertrophy" is a medical term that means the muscle is thickening, making it harder for the heart to pump blood in and out. He was offered an ICD, which delivers an electric shock to the heart if it detects an irregular heartbeat.

The device also collects hundreds of data points, all day, every day, about Campos's heart function. The information generated by his ICD could help him manage his health, but the data feed is locked down by the manufacturer. Only professional technicians and clinicians can access it, not Campos himself. Meanwhile, Campos lives in, as he puts it, "a state of constant vigilance as I adapt and change my strategies in order to manage this tricky condition." It is like driving a car in the dark, with all the lights on the dashboard out, while spectators monitor from afar, with full access to the car's data—and then cast blame when the driver crashes.

A crisis forced Campos to take action.

Prior to 2014, when the Affordable Care Act's elimination of preexisting condition restrictions went into effect, health insurance companies could refuse service to people like Campos. In 2012, he found himself without health insurance and unable to get coverage. He could not afford to get his ICD serviced and maintained, so he turned, as he says, to more subversive tactics to maintain his health.

He began looking online for a pacemaker programmer, a special computer that can adjust the settings on a live device attached to a person's heart. Their sale is understandably restricted to professionals, and Campos says, "When they show up on auction sites they are quickly flagged by the manufacturer, who demands they be pulled." He was jubilant when, after multiple tries and one failed attempt, he purchased a pacemaker programmer on May

29, 2012. Campos remembers the exact date because he kept the receipt. He paid $1,025 (plus $85 shipping and handling) for the programmer—about $4,000 less than others he had seen being sold online.

Campos traveled at his own expense from San Francisco, California, to a professional cardiac device training institute in Greenville, South Carolina, to learn how to use the programmer. As you might imagine, he was the only person in the class who planned to care for one client—himself.

Campos set up a cardiac monitoring station back home in California. He was able to buy most of the supplies, like specialized cables and thermal paper, but the next hurdle looked insurmountable. He needed old pacemakers and defibrillators to practice on. He wanted to gain confidence before tinkering with a device wired into his own heart—a potentially life-threatening activity. Where could he possibly find such rare commodities?

Once again, luck favored the resourceful. He befriended an eBay seller who seemed to have an infinite supply of used devices that, as Campos remembers, "often arrived with plenty of battery left in them and leads that appeared ripped out of someone's body." The seller, whose handle was "sleepinghearts," worked at a crematorium. Since pacemakers and defibrillators can explode when exposed to extreme heat, they must be removed before cremation. As Campos explains, "Family members are too grief-stricken and have other worries on their minds to ask for their loved one's device. So, some of them ended up on eBay and in my collection."

Campos founded the Bay Area ICD User Group to learn along with other people living with implantable cardiac devices, candidates for ICD surgery, and their friends and families. He is a Seeker, Networker, and Solver all in one, reaping the benefits of better health and sharing his insights with fellow patients, researchers, and policymakers as a participant ambassador for the All of Us research program at NIH. Few can match his tenacity, but do not believe anyone who says that patients do not want access to their own data or will not know what to do with it when they do get access. Campos and the #WeAreNotWaiting movement tell a different story.

It is wrong to cut off access to the tools people need to solve their own problems. The next chapter expands on the theme of what, besides data access, Solvers need to do their work.

Takeaways:

1. Access to one's own health data is essential to self-management of complex conditions.
2. A rebel alliance can push from the outside for change. But the patient-led revolution also needs insiders, people who follow traditional paths, in order to reach everyone.
3. Solvers can be incredibly creative and resourceful when lives are on the line.

8 TOOLS AND RESOURCES

In 1929, Werner Forssmann was a twenty-five-year-old, newly minted doctor when he began exploring ways to thread a catheter into a human heart. He was impatient to try out his idea, so, as he wrote, "After successful tests upon a cadaver, I undertook the first study on a living person, in the form of an experiment upon myself."[1] He inserted a thin surgical tube called a cannula into the plump vein on the inside of his own elbow. He then threaded a catheter, a second flexible tube, into the first one and snaked it up into the right side of his heart. He calmly walked over to the X-ray department and asked a nurse to capture an image, proving he had done it and survived. He did not wait. He acted.

Nobody would listen to Barry Marshall, MD, when he claimed that ulcers were caused by bacteria, not stress. It was too outlandish—and simple—an explanation. He could not ethically experiment on anyone but himself, so, in 1983, Marshall harvested a sample of *Helicobacter pylori* bacteria from a patient with stomach ulcers, drank it, tracked his own symptoms, proved his case, and turned the clinical understanding of ulcers upside down. Again, he did not wait. He acted.

Seven Nobel Prizes have been awarded to people who tested their ideas on themselves first. When will the first Nobel Prize be awarded to a patient-led team of Solvers?

People whose needs are not being met are both a massive market and a pool of potential inventors and innovators. We need more patients, survivors, and caregivers to connect with each other, identify challenges, get or create the tools they need, and attack problems. This chapter is about what Solvers need: communities, workspaces, and showcases.

SOLVERS NEED SEEKERS AND NETWORKERS

Jimmy Choi is an elite athlete who lives with early onset PD. Millions of people follow him on TikTok, which he mostly uses to share how-to and inspirational fitness videos. One day in December 2020, he shared a close-up video of his trembling hand trying to get a tiny pill out of a bottle. He overlaid the video with the words "Pharma executives: 'Hey! Let's make a pill for Parkinson's patients as small as F#CKIN& possible!'"

Brian Alldridge, a videographer with no special design skills, happened to see Choi's video. Alldridge had experienced short-term disability after a serious car accident in 2015, and it gave him an appreciation for the daily inconveniences that can break someone's spirit. "I'm going to solve this," he said to himself. What he realized later, though, was that his community was going to solve it.

He reshared Choi's post on his own TikTok channel with the caption, "Does someone want to make this guy a container? #3dprinting" and then set to work designing a prototype of a bottle that dispenses one pill at a time. Within a few days, thousands of people were following along, contributing ideas and offering help. TikTok's additive manufacturing community responded to Alldridge's use of the #3dprinting hashtag like it was a signal flare in the night sky.

Six months later, Alldridge's design, refined with the help of a far-flung community, was under review by the US Patent and Trademark Office. Alldridge says the 3D-printed version will always be available for free under an open license.

The right pop-up peer group met the right problem and fixed a wrong that has been vexing people with low dexterity and tremor for years. Jimmy Choi started on the far left of the needs not met spectrum, and, thanks to being a Seeker and Networker, he connected virtually with Alldridge, a Solver, and pulled himself and everyone who hears about the new pill bottle closer to the right side, where needs are met (figure 8.1).

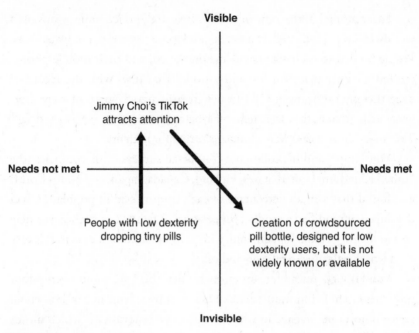

Figure 8.1
Rebel Health Matrix: Pill bottle.

LOOK FOR SOLVERS INSIDE COMMUNITIES

You might wonder how common it is for people to freelance their treatments, as Alder, Riggare, or those ALS patients did. How many people are modifying their assistive and medical devices—or inventing new ones, like the PD and diabetes communities did? How might we encourage such experimentation and help more people become Solvers?

The good news is that we are still in the early days of the patient-led revolution. We can follow the path forged by other industries that have already incorporated user-driven innovation.

Eric von Hippel is a professor at the MIT Sloan School of Management who tracks the invention and innovation happening at kitchen tables and in garages all across the world. His insights on user innovation have helped companies—and whole industries—recognize and profit from the advancements created by the people who use their products and services.

For example, 50 percent of mobile financial service innovations used worldwide were pioneered by users in developing countries, not by bankers. People needed to exchange payments on the go, and their mobile phones created a handy platform for innovation.[2] That jibes with the record of drug therapy innovation. Of 143 new treatments, 57 percent were user-generated—that is, they were new, off-label applications of an existing drug.[3] The "users" in this case were clinicians caring for patients.

Von Hippel and his colleagues conducted surveys in six countries (the United Kingdom, United States, Finland, Canada, Japan, and South Korea) and found that a small percentage of each country's adult population had developed or modified a product for personal or family use, such as a camera app to identify colors for someone who is color-blind or a coat that is easy for a wheelchair user to take on and off.

Von Hippel's research team estimates that there are about twenty-four million household innovators across all six countries. Nine in ten "household sector innovators" engage in what he calls "free innovation," which means they build and experiment in their spare time and do not actively protect their ideas from other people. Less than 10 percent of home-based innovators say they would like to develop and bring a product to market.[4]

Christiana von Hippel, a research scientist (and Eric's daughter), dug deeper into the survey data set and drew out lessons for the field of public health.[5] Household health innovators are more apt to share their ideas with peers than with clinicians or people who could commercialize new services or inventions. They are particularly likely to share with peers if they think their innovation is going to help other people and if they have an easy way to do so, such as access to social media or another network. The tremor-proof

---

Tip for Champions: Look for a Community's Assets, Not Its Deficits

Don't intervene in patient communities from a top-down, "we know best" perspective. Search first for the solutions that community members themselves have created. Find and support the Solvers.

> **Tip for Solvers: Run Before You Can Walk**
>
> If you have an idea about what people like you need, do not think to yourself, "I've got the greatest idea in the world," and then create it alone and in secret. Start building what you think should exist. Test it. Show people prototypes made out of cardboard, tape, and sticky notes. Watch to see who finds it useful. What do they find valuable? Build up those features. What do they hate—or ignore? Fix those glitches fast. If you are also a Networker, leverage the lead users in your community to get expert feedback. The ability to make constant, small improvements is an immense advantage over established companies that may be working on similar projects. Take advantage.

pill bottle innovators fit this profile, as do people who share hacks for living with low dexterity, whether because of arthritis, Moebius syndrome, or limb difference.

Solvers often can't wait to share helpful tips or creations with their peers. If they can't find an outlet, they create one, like a hashtag community on Twitter or the /r/STD subreddit. Savvy leaders tune into those conversations to learn about new business opportunities or ways to improve existing products and services.

SOLVERS TAKE RISKS

Another useful concept for understanding peer health innovation is "lead users." As Eric von Hippel defined it in 1986, lead users "face needs that will be general in a marketplace—but face them months or years before the bulk of that marketplace encounters them" and "are positioned to benefit significantly by obtaining a solution to those needs"[6] (figure 8.2).

Lead users make what they need. That simple statement glosses over the frustration and even rage an innovator feels about a tool that doesn't do its job. In the context of diabetes, "need" does not capture the exhaustion of a parent waking up every few hours to check on a child because there is no other way to mitigate the fear and real risk of them dying in their sleep from low blood sugar. Solvers invent their way out of bad situations. They take

The Lead User Curve

The curve illustrates the shape of a market trend.
Lead users have needs that are well ahead of the trend;
over time, more and more people feel the same need.

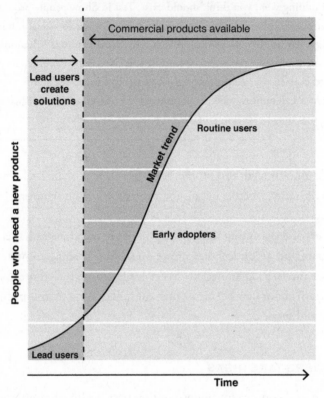

Figure 8.2
Eric von Hippel's lead user curve, recreated with permission.

risks that the rest of us would not because, well, the rest of us may not look death in the eye on a daily basis.

Dana Lewis, John Costik, and Bryan Mazlish are lead users of diabetes device innovation. The question is, will commercial manufacturers and other mainstream health-care institutions take their cues from these innovators and create new products and services for the rest of the insulin-requiring diabetes population? Or will they continue to look the other way?

Similarly, when most clinicians and researchers neglected to investigate post-viral illnesses, people with ME/CFS became lead users of patient-led research. They documented their symptoms, traded advice with each other on social platforms, and organized studies on their own. Then, when the mass-disabling event of the COVID-19 pandemic occurred, the ME/CFS patients shared their playbooks with Long COVID patients. The two groups banded together and finally got the attention of mainstream health-care leaders. The invisible became visible.

All of this illustrates the opportunities presented by the patient-led revolution. The more we can build everyone's innovation skills and increase their access to the tools and information they need to solve their own problems, the faster we will build a healthy population whose needs are met. Further, these innovators will generate breakthrough ideas for health and health care. We need to remove barriers to participation across all aspects of health innovation, from assistive and medical devices to biotechnology.

We need to unleash the lead users of health care. All those not yet being served by existing institutions, products, and services are potential innovators.

SOLVERS NEED COMMUNITIES

When people join or create a peer health community, they might be satisfied, at first, with sharing stories and advice, pleased that they have found others like themselves. Connection is a cool cloth on a hot forehead. It is a relief just to be together in community.

But then, one day, someone posts a question about a problem they can't solve. Someone else answers it. Another person adds their insights. Maybe a debate ensues. Research is done. Code is shared openly, then improved by someone else. Eventually, hopefully, the problem is solved. Together.

This creation of shared tools and assets is an essential component of a group becoming a team. As early as 1993, online culture guru Howard Rheingold observed, "Every cooperative group of people exists in the face of a competitive world because that group of people recognizes there is something valuable that they can gain only by banding together. Looking for a group's collective goods is a way of looking for the elements that bind isolated individuals into a community."[7]

In the context of health, researchers like Erin Willis have tracked how online communities transform into platforms for problem-solving. While observing members of an online arthritis support group, for example, Willis found evidence that the "microbenefits of social support or effective communication support the macrobenefit of self-management." As she writes,

> Community members collaborated to solve problems and this collective gathering and reporting of information then was applied to manage disease symptoms. The community often engaged in questioning and researching unfamiliar topics; members shared online resources and participated in discussing certain topics such as fibromyalgia, biologic medication side effects, and exercising safely. Doctors and physicians may communicate best practices of self-management behaviors to patients, but within the online health community patients "compare notes of experience" and collectively figure out the best way to manage arthritis symptoms.[8]

The question is, How to spark this transformation? When does a group become a problem-solving community?

Meeting in person is helpful, but not required. The rebel health ecosystem thrives even in times of physical isolation, like a pandemic, thanks to online collaboration platforms. This is a business opportunity as community-led innovation accelerates. We need to create more places—both virtual and physical—for people to meet, exchange ideas, and build on each other's prototypes.

SOLVERS NEED COLLABORATION PLATFORMS

Solvers thrive when they can experiment, build models, and get feedback from colleagues. They gather in places where they can meet other problem-solvers, online or offline.

Again, we can draw inspiration from product innovation scholarship. Christoph Hienerth and Christopher Lettl, professors of innovation in Germany and Austria, respectively, conducted a longitudinal research study to track what role peer communities play in developing new medical and sporting equipment. They identified the three primary requirements for user innovation to occur:[9]

- Users have a high need for innovations
- Communities exist
- The means of production are available to both users and manufacturers

The rebel health alliance has demonstrated or built the first two requirements. There is a burgeoning marketplace for health-care innovation by and for patients and caregivers—and Seekers show that there is an appetite for more. Networkers have built thousands of thriving communities. The next step is to upgrade those communities from meeting spaces to collaboration platforms.

Solvers need a place to pool their ideas and debate, asynchronously, about findings and next steps. That often happens by email, on social media, or on other platforms that were not built for long-term collaboration, like Facebook. A few companies, like PatientsLikeMe (PLM), Inspire, StuffThatWorks, and Hive Networks (a company I advise), have built platforms to offer health data tracking tools, secure data storage, and threaded discussion boards. Between 2004 and 2018, for example, PLM collected more than forty-three million real-world data points from 650,000 members of the platform whose observations spanned 2,900 health conditions.[10] The collaboration platform market is ripe for investment as patient-led innovation grows.

SOLVERS NEED LABS AND MAKERSPACES

Some Solvers need to work with specialized tools and to get expert guidance as they improve their inventions. This is the third requirement of user innovation: access to the means of production. Here are examples of leading-edge initiatives to democratize discovery and invention:

Labs: Research-grade tools are no longer limited to university and corporate labs thanks to community biolabs and the decentralized science movement. Some organizations, such as Biocurious and the Baltimore Underground

Science Space, aim to allow people to safely and affordably explore, while others, like Alexandria Launch Labs and BioLabs, focus on launching start-ups.

In addition to physical laboratory equipment, citizen-scientists benefit from access to research tools like protocols and standards for conducting experiments. Online communities of self-experimenters have created new models for discovery. By sharing their practices, they create a parallel structure that is outside but adjacent to traditional science.

For example, John Bailey and Joanna Kempner, sociologists at Rutgers University, chronicled the work of a group of citizen-scientists engaged in drug development using psychedelic mushrooms.[11] "Clusterbusters," a non-profit focused on the alleviation of cluster headaches, developed a standardized protocol for acquiring, preparing, and testing microdoses of psilocybin at home. A key element of their success was upgrading their equipment, using laboratory-grade scales capable of measuring milligrams instead of standard kitchen scales. By organizing their own studies, they pulled themselves out of the lower-left quadrant of the Rebel Health Matrix. Participants found relief and scientists in the biomedical mainstream found new pathways to treatments that work.

Makerspaces: Community makerspaces are one example of physical workshops where people can rent or borrow tools, learn new skills, and find collaborators. Inventors, entrepreneurs, and artists are the traditional customers for makerspaces, but an organization called MakerHealth is bringing the concept to health care.

Anna Young and Jose Gomez-Marquez cofounded MakerHealth to expand the work they were doing at the MIT Little Devices Lab, which focuses on DIY health technologies from around the world. They built the first makerspace in a hospital in 2015 and have created a virtual program, too, furthering their "mission to democratize the skills and tools to create and invent the things you can hold in your hand." An innovation that a nurse, patient, or family caregiver comes up with on the fly to help one person can now be prototyped, tested, and deployed at scale thanks to MakerHealth's training, tools, and online community. It is a model for how to help Solvers.

For example, an intensive-care unit nurse used a sewing machine from her hospital's makerspace to make a head support device for a patient on life support. This patient is a new mother and, when she was discharged from the hospital and into a rehabilitation center, she worked with an occupational therapist to create a custom strength-building device so she could begin to carry her baby. About one-quarter of the projects at that hospital are collaborations between clinicians and patients.

MakerHealth has also worked with patient associations, such as the Scleroderma Foundation in Massachusetts and an elder learning center in Texas, to teach people prototyping skills. Participants then design and make personalized solutions for clinical and everyday challenges.

Gokul Krishnan, another Champion of patient-led innovation, created the organization Maker Therapy to bring tools and materials to children and teens in pediatric clinical settings. Since young patients are often confined to their rooms, Krishnan designed a mobile cart with all the materials and tools a kid could use to create, for example, a pill cup that lights up so a patient can see it in the dark. It also rotates, for no reason other than it was designed by an eight-year-old who thought it would be cool.

Everyone is a potential inventor, and initiatives like MakerHealth and Maker Therapy show how we can bring that spirit to health care. We need makerspaces designed for both clinicians and patients in every hospital,

---

Tip for Solvers: Look for Partners Who Have Something to Prove

The dominant player in a market may not be the one you want to approach with your idea. If you are hoping to catch the attention of a hospital leader, for example, don't pitch the most famous facility in your area. Reach out to smaller, regional hospitals since they often have more to prove and may be more willing to take on a patient-led initiative. Similarly, device makers who command the majority of their market may not think they need input from patient-led teams. That's an opening that another company can step into. When it comes to medical specialties, multiple Solvers advised starting in pediatrics, a smaller field that is hungry for improvement. There is more room for trying something different.

but even better in settings that are accessible to everyone who wants to be a Solver.

SOLVERS NEED A SHOWCASE

Once a Solver has created something they think is useful, they need a place to share it with a broader network of potential users. Again, this happens on social media, but the impact is diluted because there is no central repository for peer-produced innovations. An international nonprofit based in Portugal fills that gap for devices, apps, and therapies. Patient Innovation (patient -innovation.com) "connects patients and caregivers, and enables the sharing of their solutions. If not shared, these strategies, treatments, devices, and knowledge would probably remain unknown to many patients, not fulfilling their potential to change the lives of others."[12]

The site features over 1,000 innovations shared by patients, caregivers, and collaborators across a range of about 260 health conditions or challenges. The top five conditions with solutions on the platform include physical disability, paraplegia, cerebral palsy, blindness, and autism. The organization's research has shown that people with nascent ideas who have been able to interact with peer health innovators are more likely to create prototypes,[13] so Patient Innovation has sponsored or sent mentors to make-a-thons all over Europe. The site serves to both organize the patient-innovator community and act as an intermediary, connecting Solvers with Champions, who can help bring new products to market.

Solvers need more platforms to share their innovations, whether they are assistive devices and other hardware, or less tangible treatment, process, and service delivery improvements. And Solvers need more institutions to sponsor in-person events so they can gather and learn from each other. Society needs this too. Solvers often serve the needs of people who are invisible to mainstream health care—that lower-left quadrant of the Rebel Health Matrix (figure 8.3).

Savvy Champions can monitor and invest in the solutions that Solvers create, helping them to reach new audiences and markets. Because while

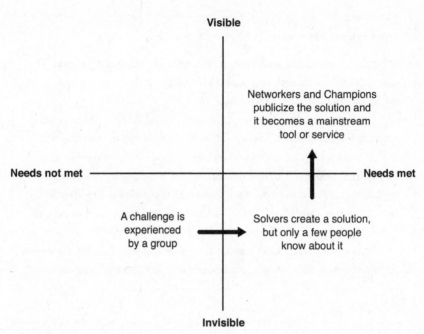

Figure 8.3
Rebel Health Matrix: Solvers need Networkers and Champions.

having a personally life-changing idea is great, getting access to resources to turn it into a world-changing idea is even better.

Innovation is more often a group project than an individual achievement. Magic happens when people can meet, exchange ideas, and build on one another's concepts. Proximity—sometimes literally bumping into people who can help answer your latest, burning question—creates a constant conversation among Seekers, Networkers, Solvers, and Champions. That can happen in physical spaces, such as conference hallways or start-up incubators, or in online communities.

Tip for Solvers: Pitch Better

Solvers need resources, which means you need investors and partners. You need to learn how to pitch your ideas to both believers, who are excited about the future, and skeptics, who are not.

A one-size-fits-all approach will not work. Instead, create two completely different pitches. For the evangelized, paint a grand vision that emphasizes the excitement of your innovation and the radical change it represents. For the skeptics, reassure them that this innovation is important, but in line with everything they have been doing. It won't take them long to incorporate the change into their workflow. Create an easy way for them to see how partnering with you would benefit them.

Create two pitch decks—one for the evangelists and the other for skeptics. Before every meeting, do your research so you know which pitch to use.

Takeaways:

1. The patient-led revolution is aligned with the concept of "user innovation."
2. Solvers need access to each other, to information, to data, and to workspaces.

9 CHAMPIONS

On August 29, 2005, Nick Gautreaux was shocked by the images of the water rising in New Orleans, just two hours east of where he lives in Lafayette, Louisiana.[1] Hurricane Katrina had overwhelmed the city's flood protection structures and 80 percent of New Orleans was underwater.

Gautreaux, a Louisiana state senator at the time, immediately started making plans to help rescue people. He reached out to his Senate colleague Walter Boasso to see what he could learn about the situation in a hard-hit area of New Orleans, St. Bernard Parish. Boasso texted back, "My people are dying. Please send help." Gautreaux replied, "Don't worry. Help is on the way."

Gautreaux made his appeal on the local news: if you have a boat, come to the Acadiana Mall on Johnston Street by 5 a.m. the next day. From there, he planned to caravan to New Orleans and start rescuing people wherever they found them. Hundreds of people from all over south Louisiana showed up on August 30 with boats of every shape and size. Gautreaux grabbed a bullhorn, not to rally the troops but to warn them: "This is the deal. If you're afraid to see death, don't come. If you're afraid to see a dead body floating in the water, don't come. . . . If you're not used to the smell of death, don't come with us." Not a single person left.

These boaters did not wait for the blessing of any authorities—and in some cases, they defied them, heading out into the flooded city of New Orleans against the advice of officials guarding the perimeter. They deputized themselves and set out to rescue as many people as they could, using cell phones and broadcast radio to organize a distributed response. They became known as the

Cajun Navy for their Louisiana roots and they (along with new recruits) have answered the call to service in many disasters since then. They react fast, before the federal government can get to people, and they save lives.

The Cajun Navy inspired Craig Fugate, former head of the Federal Emergency Management Agency (FEMA), to rethink the role of the public in a disaster. Instead of seeing the public as a liability, he realized FEMA should see them as a resource.[2] Neighbors, family members, and bystanders are the real first responders at the scene of a disaster. That realization fueled FEMA's "whole-community response" strategy, which recognizes that locals know better than anyone what people need and how to get it to them.

That shift in perspective—to see the public as a resource—is fundamental to the patient-led revolution. While not a story about health care, the Cajun Navy is an example of the grassroots cooperative approach that Solvers use. When FEMA began incorporating distributed, civilian-led rescue teams into the federal government's emergency response plan, the agency became a Champion, a mainstream institution that can help take a scrappy peer-led idea to scale.

We need all hands on deck to change the health-care system for the better. This chapter is about how Seekers, Networkers, and Solvers can find Champions—and vice versa.

AGAINST THE ODDS

Here's how the Cajun Navy illustrates the archetypes of the patient-led revolution (figure 9.1):

Seekers. People's needs are not being met. They seek help. (Picture people standing on rooftops, surrounded by water.)

Networkers. People find each other and form a group. They communicate with each other and pool resources. They are not alone. (People call and text the locations of those who are trapped to rescuers outside the flood zone.)

Solvers. Someone suggests a new way to approach a problem. (Locals with boats take to the water to start rescuing everyone they can find.)

Champions. People with access to resources fast-track innovations. (FEMA creates the strategy of a "whole-community response" to disasters.)

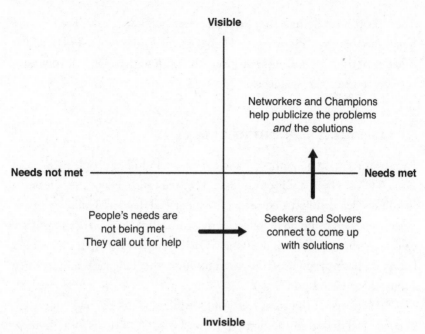

Visible

Networkers and Champions
help publicize the problems
and the solutions

Needs not met —————————————————— **Needs met**

People's needs are
not being met
They call out for help

Seekers and Solvers
connect to come up
with solutions

Invisible

Figure 9.1
Rebel Health Matrix: Cajun Navy.

In a health-care context, the innovation might be a new treatment, practice, approach, or device. People in need think the idea has promise, so they invest their own time and resources into designing, building, testing, and refining the innovation. The group becomes a team. They start adding members with new skills and capabilities. They create and share their working prototype. Those who are lucky enough to hear about the innovation have the chance to adopt it.

Lots of Solvers stop here. Maybe they have solved their own problem and are satisfied. Maybe they run out of money. Maybe they grow frustrated with a lack of progress. Maybe the group disperses once the excitement of creating something new has passed. Maybe they don't see a pathway toward further publicizing the innovation or they are not interested in taking it to scale.

But there are teams who decide to go for it, against the odds. They take chances that other people would not because they do not see another choice.

Their people are dying. They see their peers stranded, exhausted, losing hope, and they say, "Don't worry. Help is on the way." We need to build the capacity of the peer health innovation ecosystem so that every worthy team survives to reach the next level.

BUILDING A RAFT OUT OF DATA

Faced with a flood of confusion and denial, a handful of people living with Long COVID built a raft out of data. Like the Cajun Navy, they created a distributed leadership structure for the Patient-Led Research Collaborative—five people who could fill in for each other since all of them were ailing. They called on other members of the Long COVID diaspora to help translate their survey on prolonged COVID symptoms into other languages and recruit a robust sample of respondents.

Within weeks, the volunteers, often while sick in bed, had conceived, created, and delivered the first report on Long COVID. Suddenly these patients were briefing officials at the WHO, the CDC, and the NIH. In the United Kingdom, their findings were cited both by Parliament and the National Institute for Health and Care Excellence. In a world hungry for data about this mysterious phenomenon, officials devoured the Patient-Led Research Collaborative's survey results and became Champions of their work.

A crisis created the conditions for these institutions to look outside the usual channels for insight. A patient-led research team delivered what the world needed: a new way to collect real-time epidemiological data. Long COVID patients' own voices were heard on the international stage.

PATIENT-LED CLINICAL RESEARCH

Cancer is another personal hurricane that jolts people into action.

Michael Katz, diagnosed with multiple myeloma in 1990, was dropped into the dark maze of rare cancer. A finding of terminal, incurable illness is a shocking event for anyone, but perhaps particularly for a thirty-seven-year-old enjoying his three children and a career as a global management consultant. A fellow patient, who had been diagnosed with this same cancer of the bone marrow just three years before, guided Katz to the information he needed to map out his own treatment choices. He vowed to do the same for other people.

Katz volunteered to help a patient-led organization, the International Myeloma Foundation (IMF), upgrade its patient database and laboratory results tracker. He threw himself into advocacy and connecting with other patients, peer-to-peer, through both IMF and ACOR, the same collection of online communities that helped Dave deBronkart when he was diagnosed with kidney cancer.

Through this work, Katz saw that cancer patients were frustrated. Nobody with real power was focused on the problems they wanted to solve. It was up to them to save their people. Like so many rebels before them, patients deputized themselves.

Over the course of a decade, Katz rose to become the chair of the Patient Representative Committee for the Eastern Cooperative Oncology Group (ECOG), which conducts multicenter clinical trials for cancer research. He sat at the table with clinicians and scientists as an equal, advocating for the investigation of questions that patients wanted answered. This is a model for other researchers to follow when working with patients.

In 2002, S. Vincent Rajkumar, MD, chair of ECOG and an expert on blood cancer at the Mayo Clinic, was excited about the prospect of testing new drugs for multiple myeloma. Katz pushed back. That is not what patients want, Katz said, adding that "all these new drugs don't help if patients cannot take them." Too many people were unable to survive the established first-line treatment, dexamethasone, which was being given at a high dose by default because nobody had ever tested its effectiveness at lower doses.

The rest of the committee was skeptical. Why test the dosing of a drug that worked to kill cancer cells and was widely accepted by clinicians?

"To us the idea seemed destined to fail," Rajkumar recalls. "It seemed so boring. We had waited 40 years for new drugs and Mike wants us to test dex dosing! However, we respected Mike. We knew he was aware of what patients were going through. We saw 100–200 myeloma patients a year. He interacted with thousands. He was also leading meetings of support group leaders who were leading meetings with lots of other myeloma patients." The clinicians convinced their institutional sponsors to try Katz's idea.

Patients were so eager to participate in the clinical trial for lower-dose dexamethasone that all the spots were filled in record time—faster than any other national, cooperative multiple myeloma trial. And, as it turns out, patients were right to push for the change. At the one-year mark, 96 percent of participants on the low-dose regimen were alive, compared with 87 percent of those on the high-dose, standard-of-care treatment. Serious side effects, like blood clots, were also reduced among those on low-dose dexamethasone, which has become the new standard. And, just as Katz had predicted, using a lower dose of dex has allowed oncologists to build new drug combinations.

When the randomized trial of high-dose versus low-dose dexamethasone was published in *The Lancet Oncology*, it became one of the most cited myeloma papers ever.[3] And it is thanks to a patient who heard his community crying out that their people were dying. He was able to answer, "Don't worry. Help is on the way."

When Katz was diagnosed, he was a Seeker—terrified, alone, but determined to find the best information he could. He quickly became a Networker, using online platforms to help myeloma patients and researchers connect with information and with each other. He rebuilt IMF's patient database and started the myeloma group on ACOR, gathering insights from thousands of patients about their treatments. Finally, acknowledged as an expert in his own right, he was invited by the leaders of ECOG and NCI to serve as an advisor. Crucially, the scientists and clinicians listened to him. They championed his proposal for a study based on the insights gleaned from the patient-led myeloma groups.

Michael Katz died in 2015 from complications related to multiple myeloma, twenty-four years after his diagnosis. His legacy endures because other patients, clinicians, and researchers have followed the path he forged. Dr. Rajkumar shared the story on Twitter years later to attract attention to Katz's accomplishments, to show colleagues how powerful it can be to listen to and work with patients. In the patient-led revolution model, Katz is a Seeker-Networker and Rajkumar is a Champion. They bridged the gap between what patients need and what scientists and clinicians are able to deliver. They showed that it is a competitive advantage for clinicians, researchers, and funders to work with patients.

By doing so, Katz and Rajkumar followed a path that was forged many years before by a small group of visionary health-care leaders.

VISIONARIES

In chapter 4, I pointed to the *Whole Earth Catalog* as an early prototype of the internet, connecting people with specialized information, tools, and, crucially, each other. Tom Ferguson, MD, was the first medical editor for the *Whole Earth Catalog* and an early contributor to online communities like the WELL. He was a tireless advocate for people gaining access to the information and tools they needed to take care of themselves, online or offline. Like Katz, he lived with multiple myeloma, and he applied the principles of being an engaged patient to his own treatment, as well as spreading the gospel to others. And he wasn't alone in this work.

One of Ferguson's mentors and colleagues, Warner Slack, MD, was a visionary "cybermedicine" pioneer who taught at Harvard Medical School. As far back as 1976, Dr. Slack declared, "We should try to make it easy for patients to care for themselves when they want to. Our goal with the computer is to help patients help themselves."[4] In a later article, he wrote that "communication between patients and doctors should not be used to persuade patients to do what physicians want them to do; rather, it should be used to outline the possible plans of action, so that patients can decide clinical matters for themselves."[5]

Another pioneer Champion of the patient-led revolution, Kate Lorig, DrPH, created and studied peer-led health education for people living with arthritis in the early 1980s at Stanford.[6] Unlike many conditions, arthritis waxes and wanes, requiring each person to adapt their exercise, rest, and even medications to their needs on a particular day.[7] Lorig and her colleagues showed that asking someone to become an active participant in a peer-led program, not simply a recipient of information, is essential to reaping the benefits of self-empowerment and agency. The effects of this psychological shift—less pain, fewer clinical visits, and cost savings—are sustained over years.

In 1984, Donald A. B. Lindberg, MD, then the newly appointed director of the US National Library of Medicine (NLM), authorized the creation of a user-friendly portal for the library's vast resources. The NLM aimed to open its archives to everyone who had access to a computer; in a nod to the counterculture that inspired the information revolution, the new system was called "Grateful Med."

It took a bold leap of imagination to foresee that regular people would be interested in accessing the NLM's electronic archives. A national poll conducted around that time found that only 10 percent of US adults said they had a home computer and, of those, 14 percent said they used a modem to send and receive information over telephone lines, which meant that less than 2 percent of US adults had access to the internet in the 1980s. But Ferguson, Slack, Lorig, Lindberg, and others were building not for what was, but what could be: a possible future in which people researched their own conditions and treatments online, shared what they found with peers, and participated in managing their own health. These visionary clinicians were Champions of the patient-, survivor-, and caregiver-led revolution.

STRENGTH IN NUMBERS

More than any other condition group, the DOC typifies health care's Cajun Navy. Nobody was focused on the problems they wanted to solve, so the

---

Tip for Champions: Create Opportunities for Scale

If you spot a rebel health team that has executed a successful pilot or launched a new product or service in a small market, recruit them to your incubator, start-up accelerator, or other existing structure that helps entrepreneurs scale. Innovators make faster progress when they can pour their ideas into a ready container. A Champion can help Solvers wrap a business reason around an idea and help it succeed.

DOC set about solving them on their own. They rallied together in person and on social media. They liberated their own device data. And they built what they needed to save lives. This scrappy band of patients and caregivers could not be ignored. They were plucking people out of the rising waters of diabetes and giving them hope.

But the water creeps up slowly with a chronic condition like diabetes, so slowly that it doesn't appear to be a crisis—until it is your friend or family member who is trapped and begging for help.

Like the Cajun Navy and the Patient-Led Research Collaborative, the DOC's strength is that no one person is in charge. Individuals have done great—even heroic—things in the push toward improvement of diabetes devices, platforms, and treatments, but the real credit goes to the collective.

Here's the story of how a Champion emerged from within a community and rallied its members to rise up and demand change.

AN OPEN LETTER

In 2007, Amy Tenderich, founder of DiabetesMine, used her skills as a Networker to shine a spotlight on her community's needs. She wrote an open letter to Steve Jobs, the CEO of Apple, since he was famous for demanding seamless user experiences and beautiful design.[8] Tenderich pointed out that "medical device manufacturers are stuck in a bygone era; they continue to design these products in an engineering-driven, physician-centered bubble. They have not yet grasped the concept that medical devices are also life devices, and therefore need to feel good and look good for the patients using them 24/7, in addition to keeping us alive."

Her letter got picked up and amplified, first by the DOC, then by the technology press, and finally by mainstream media outlets. The idea for user-centered diabetes device design went from a conversation among Networkers and Solvers to being noticed by potential Champions.

Tenderich and her team responded by organizing a formal design challenge in 2008, calling on people all over the world to reimagine tools to improve life with diabetes. As far as she knows, this was the first-ever crowdsourcing innovation competition aimed at a health-care challenge, and certainly the first

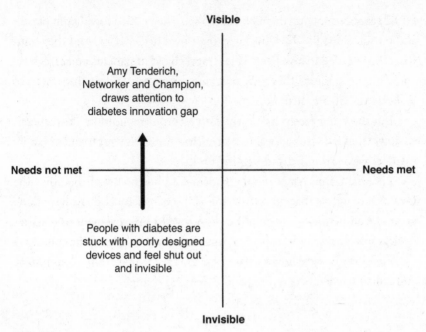

Visible

Amy Tenderich,
Networker and Champion,
draws attention to
diabetes innovation gap

Needs not met ⟵⟶ Needs met

People with diabetes are
stuck with poorly designed
devices and feel shut out
and invisible

Invisible

Figure 9.2
Rebel Health Matrix: DiabetesMine.

to be led by a patient influencer. People submitted hundreds of ideas for new products, from basics like more stylish and useful carrying cases for diabetes management supplies to sophisticated medical device prototypes and apps. Tenderich stepped into the role of Champion, infusing the field of patient-led diabetes innovation with resources and visibility (figure 9.2).

WE ARE NOT WAITING

After running that competition successfully for four years, the DiabetesMine team began convening annual meetings of patients, caregivers, clinicians, entrepreneurs, and designers to talk about how to innovate in the high-stakes world of diabetes. Every time one group tried to blame another for slowing down progress, Tenderich made sure to invite the scapegoats to the next meeting. She created an environment in which Solvers could meet with each other *and* with potential Champions for their ideas.

Soon, every stakeholder was coming to the DiabetesMine meetings. In 2012, three FDA officials attended the DiabetesMine Innovation Summit as did the CEO and the chief scientific and medical officer of the American Diabetes Association. Regulators were talking directly with patients, hackers were sitting in the same room with device manufacturers, and, in 2013, just six months after John Costik freed his son's device data, a working group gathered to hash out what the DOC could do with this new resource: direct access to their own health data. The group decided to move forward whether the powers that be were ready or not. As the activists put it, "We are not waiting." It was at that meeting that the phrase became a rallying cry, connecting people across the world on social platforms. It helped Seekers, Networkers, and Solvers raise the visibility of their cause and draw the attention of potential Champions.

The people who collaborated to build Nightscout, the DIY diabetes surveillance system, made their code open-source and published a step-by-step guide and how-to videos (along with warnings that the system is "highly experimental. Not intended for therapy. Use at your own risk. Intended only as an investigational and educational tool to learn about this technology").[9] Hundreds, even thousands of people benefited from this small-group problem-solving.

We Are Not Waiting

#WeAreNotWaiting to bridge disconnected data islands.
#WeAreNotWaiting for competitors to cooperate.
#WeAreNotWaiting for regulators to regulate.
#WeAreNotWaiting for device manufacturers to innovate.
#WeAreNotWaiting for payers to pay.
#WeAreNotWaiting for others to decide if, when, and how we access and use
    data from our own bodies.
#WeAreNotWaiting to build applications that focus on design and usability.
#WeAreNotWaiting for the cure.

—from a #WeAreNotWaiting Diabetes DIY movement manifesto

What happened next is even more extraordinary. The patient-led, peer-to-peer innovation kept spreading. The FDA and device companies took notes. And in 2015, Dexcom, one of the major manufacturers of diabetes management devices, responded to the market demand it was seeing in these peer-to-peer networks and created a CGM with a share function that can send data to a smartphone.

But the diabetes rebel alliance of Seekers, Networkers, and Solvers was not satisfied. They wanted a way for all diabetes devices to share data. They needed a trustworthy ambassador to broker a deal with leaders who hold the purse strings and the power.

AMBASSADOR

Howard Look is a technology executive who works across sectors and translates geek-speak to the C-suite. He led software teams at TiVo, Pixar, Linden Lab, and Amazon, building his knowledge of user experience, cloud-connected devices, and open-source code until the moment it all came together in service of fixing the technology that keeps his daughter, Katie, alive.

In 2011, when Katie, then eleven, was diagnosed with insulin-requiring diabetes, she and her family were sucked into the Seeker vortex, navigating a new landscape of illness and risk. Howard Look dove into online conversations about how to manage the devices that ruled their lives, and, once he understood the scope of the challenge, left his job building consumer electronic devices at Amazon and founded a nonprofit, Tidepool, in 2013. He was motivated by love for Katie and anger at a system that repelled change. "Innovation in the medical device world doesn't have to go at a snail's pace," he says, and he set out to prove it. The first person he hired was Ben West.

Tidepool's initial goal was to liberate data from diabetes devices, to make it actionable and useful. By positioning themselves as a radically transparent nonprofit, they could take the high road and say to companies, "It's not your data, it's not our data; it's the patients' data, and we're here to make sure that they get access to it."

Tidepool succeeded in changing most companies' lock-it-up data policies. Those who didn't comply with their requests soon found out that PWDs were not waiting any longer for permission. "We reverse-engineered the Medtronic pump protocol and got the data out anyway," says Look. "The FDA was fine with that. We published the code, and we were the only software that allows you to see Medtronic pump data and Dexcom CGM data. That is still true today."

Once they succeeded in creating a data platform, Tidepool took on a more audacious quest: seeking FDA approval for an app to automate insulin dosing. It would be an official version of what had been created by the thousands of do-it-yourselfers who looped together their devices to create a homemade artificial pancreas. Unfortunately, many people who want to loop are too nervous to attempt the installation on their own or are told by their clinicians that they will be dropped as patients if they even try a non-FDA-approved protocol.

Tidepool took the open-source code written by the diabetes rebel alliance and created something that can, with an access code prescribed by a clinician, be downloaded from the app store, installed on a smartphone, and used in conjunction with certain approved devices. It legitimizes the underground movement for change. In a milestone for patient-led initiatives, Tidepool Loop received FDA approval in January 2023.

Look is a Networker, an insider-outsider, able to pool the resources necessary for systemic change. He seized the opportunity to make his daughter's life better and then expanded his scope to improve the lives of everyone with insulin-requiring diabetes. A consummate ambassador, Look credits the community that rebelled against the status quo and built what they needed to save their own lives. They freed the data, wrote the code, and made the crucial choice to publish it using an open-source license so that anyone and everyone can use it and improve it.

WHOLE-COMMUNITY RESPONSE

The DOC created its own solutions and revealed not only an opportunity for better management of the disease but also new business opportunities for both established players and new entrants. The ensuing explosion of patient-led innovation has inspired institutions to start thinking differently about every aspect of living with diabetes.

Prize competitions yielded promising new ideas, like voice-activated diabetes education on smart speakers. Patient-led developers created new solutions like One Drop, a diabetes management system, and mySugr, a coaching app that has been acquired by Roche Diabetes Care.

Thanks to a partnership with Abbott, a Fortune 500 company, Bigfoot Biomedical gained FDA approval for a diabetes management system that integrates a continuous glucose monitoring system with a reusable smart cap for an insulin pen, a device that is more widely used than a pump. The system provides an insulin dose recommendation based on a doctor's instructions, minimizing the guesswork involved in daily life with insulin-requiring diabetes.

Each of these initiatives is an example of a team of Solvers finding Champions to invest in their ideas. So how do we replicate this whole-community response for other health conditions? Let's review the formula.

The diabetes rebel alliance gathered first online and then in person (Networkers emerged). It was catalytic to have that many diabetes hackers and pioneers communicating with each other, naming the problems and formulating solutions (Solvers emerged).

Then the suits showed up, invited by Amy Tenderich, a Champion who arose from within the patient-led community. The diabetes rebels started talking directly with leaders from pharmaceutical and device companies, the FDA, and the national diabetes advocacy groups. They learned from each other about where their missions overlapped and where they diverged. And the suits listened. They didn't agree with everything that every activist said or did. But some leaders worked with the rebels, and together, they infused the space with resources: funding, media attention, regulatory guidance, and technical know-how. A grassroots movement led by patients and caregivers changed the trajectory of diabetes care innovation.

To become Champions, people in mainstream institutions must be able to spot where their goals match those of a team of Solvers. Then the Champions can equip the Solvers with what they need, such as access to labs, manufacturing facilities, and marketing support.

As Gary Wolf, the personal science expert, put it, "Patients who have had to take charge of their own community building and data gathering efforts often do so because they are sick and therefore very motivated to make and contribute to discoveries. This is a source of innovation and leadership, but without institutional support most of these projects will not realize their potential over the long term." We cannot ask unpaid volunteers working part time to be responsible for systemic change. Champions must find and support them.

The next chapter is an illustration of why—and how to make it happen.

Takeaways:

1. Seekers, Networkers, and Solvers should be seen as valuable resources, not passive patients or consumers.
2. It is a competitive advantage to partner with Solvers.
3. Ambassadors—Networkers with credibility among both rebels and suits—can help connect patient-led teams with Champions.

10 MISSION ALIGNMENT

Fran Visco, a partner in a Philadelphia law firm, was diagnosed with breast cancer in 1987 and, shortly afterward, started volunteering for a local patient navigation organization. Four years later, she was part of the start-up phase of what would become the National Breast Cancer Coalition (NBCC). Medicine was still a "patients keep out" club, and NBCC decided to disrupt that narrative. Borrowing tactics from radical movements of the past, NBCC became the ACT UP of breast cancer. Like the AIDS activists, breast cancer patients forcefully confronted scientific gatekeepers on behalf of all those who have died—and will die—of the disease they share. Their goal is systemic change.

NBCC found an ally in Senator Tom Harkin of Iowa, whose two sisters died of breast cancer, and in 1992, Congress appropriated $210 million of the Defense Department's budget for breast cancer research. Such funds would normally go to NCI but the director had indicated that patients would not be welcome in scientific meetings. The NBCC wanted a seat at the table when the money was doled out, so Visco and her team worked with congressional staff to divert the windfall to the US Army's medical research program, supervised by Major General Richard Travis.[1]

Staying close to the problem being solved is part of the military's playbook. Travis had met with Visco and assured her that patient advocates were not only welcome but also essential partners in understanding and prioritizing breast cancer research questions.[2] Travis saw opportunities that other leaders had missed. He put patients and family caregivers on the team, unlocked new funding for his program, and became a Champion of the patient-led revolution.

This chapter is about how leaders can become Champions and help Seekers, Networkers, and Solvers break new trails through the permafrost of the status quo. Savvy Champions partner with on-the-ground experts to co-produce health care, whether they are creating a new product or improving a service. Champions create pathways both inside and outside their organizations for innovators with fresh ideas. Champions find and support the best solutions, even when they come from unusual sources.

CHAMPIONS NEED TO ALIGN WITH OUTSIDE INNOVATORS

When patient advocates recognized that they were not welcome at NCI, Fran Visco and her colleagues did not give up. They networked their way to Major General Travis, the Champion who said yes. Both NBCC and the US Army medical research team got what they wanted: access to new funding and to each other.

Under this Major General's leadership, the Department of Defense designed a program to include patients, survivors, and family caregivers in the scientific review process for all of their medical research programs. Over two thousand people have participated as reviewers since the program's launch.

NBCC members honed their skills as Networkers, building the reach of their local chapters, while Visco and her team maintained their laser focus on finding and supporting worthy clinical trials. Thanks to the combined strengths of their grassroots organizers and powerful leaders, NBCC enrolled potential trial participants much faster than any clinical center could at the time—a competitive advantage for researchers since nearly one in five clinical trials for cancer do not meet their recruitment targets using traditional methods.[3]

Genentech, for example, partnered with activists, including Visco and NBCC, to help with the oversight and logistics of a broad-based clinical trial that resulted in the development of Herceptin, a breakthrough treatment for one type of breast cancer. Just as the ECOG had listened to Michael Katz, reaping the benefits of his work as a Seeker-Networker, Genentech learned from breast cancer Networkers who spread the word faster and more effectively than professional staff ever could.

Champions need to find alignment between an institution's goals and the mission of outside innovators. Look for the Seekers, Networkers, and Solvers whose ideas for change mesh with your own plans. Partner with them.

CHAMPIONS NEED GUIDELINES FOR ETHICAL ENGAGEMENT

Champions who come from within patient-led groups, like Amy Tenderich, are likely to approach partnerships with Seekers, Networkers, and Solvers with respect at the core of every conversation. But even they, along with Champions from outside the community, benefit from reminders and guidelines for sharing power. Foundational work on collaborative frameworks and readiness has been done by groups like Genetic Alliance, the Patient-Centered Outcomes Research Institute, FasterCures, the Council of Medical Specialty Societies, and the Patient-Led Research Collaborative.[4] New frontiers of research and discovery demand new ethical guidelines.[5] Champions should educate themselves and encourage partners on all sides to learn more about inclusive and principled engagement.

At a minimum, patients, survivors, and caregivers should understand what they are being asked to do, be given opportunities to contribute at the design stage (and not asked only to react to a finished product), and have access to the outcome of the work being done with their help, whether it is a drug, device, service, or publication. Champions should look for ways to reduce burdens of time, stress, and cost, particularly when patients, survivors, and caregivers are being asked to participate in research studies.[6]

Champions can also work with an insider-outsider like Jen Horonjeff, founder and CEO of Savvy Cooperative. She helps match patients, survivors, and caregivers with companies developing products or services for their specific groups. A patient advocate herself, Horonjeff tells companies that they will "pay now or pay later" for straight talk from people in their target market. By investing in and learning from patient-led communities, companies are more likely to avoid the later expense of a failed product launch or amendment to a clinical trial protocol.[7]

CHAMPIONS NEED TO IDENTIFY AND EXPOSE BLIND SPOTS

Corporations and government agencies with multibillion-dollar budgets generally do not pay attention to the inventions that people are prototyping at home and sharing online.

This is a blind spot. Why? People who live with chronic health conditions or physical challenges rely on medical and assistive devices day in and day out. They bend tools until they break and then use what they learn to make better ones. They know what they need better than anyone else. They are the lead users of the hardware of health care.

As the chief technology officer of the US Department of HHS, I was a Champion for outside innovators who wanted to contribute to the mission of improving the health and safety of all Americans. One of my initiatives focused on patient-led medical and assistive device innovation. I needed a quick way to illustrate the difference between developing a highly regulated, complex, and expensive device (like a pacemaker) and the simpler, low-cost devices that I had seen in my fieldwork in patient communities (like the dexterity hacks used by people with Moebius syndrome or Parkinson's).

A simple 2×2 matrix fit the bill. The top of the vertical axis was labeled "high barriers to entry" (meaning that prototypes are costly, and devices are highly regulated and require access to highly specialized expertise). At the bottom were "low barriers to entry" (meaning that someone could make a prototype at very low cost with household items and no technical know-how). The far left of the horizontal axis was labeled "$N = 1$" (meaning that the solution would be tailored for one person or a small group of people). At the far right was the infinity symbol (meaning that the solution potentially has universal appeal or usefulness; figure 10.1).

This 2×2 became my calling card. Some people grasped what I was trying to say immediately—and indeed, were way ahead of me, such as those who worked in emergency response or aging-related disability. They had seen the power of low-cost, highly customizable innovations and were

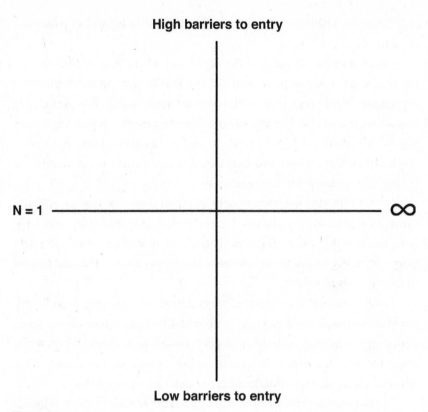

Figure 10.1
Invent Health Matrix.

ready to become Champions, opening up pathways for outside innovators to contribute to their work.

Dava Newman, then the deputy administrator at NASA, was an eager collaborator, ready to dive into a discussion about hardware innovation in low-resource environments like space or a hurricane-damaged city. She could see what I saw.

One day in 2016 I met with Robert Califf, MD, the commissioner of the FDA, to talk about the potential of patient-led collaboration around the hardware of health care. As a cardiologist, Califf has deep expertise in the medical device space, and as commissioner, he oversaw the FDA's Center for Devices and Radiological Health. I felt like I was about to explain batting practice to Joe DiMaggio. But I set up an easel with a big pad of paper and drew my 2×2.

I started to list examples of devices in each of the four quadrants—an innovative coronary stent or artificial eye lens in the top right quadrant (expensive, highly regulated, with universal application). Big money, big impact on the world. The top-left quadrant (expensive, highly regulated, highly individualized devices) is where we'd put a custom lower-limb prosthetic. Intensively tested and engineered because there is no margin for failure. You do not want someone to fall.

Next, I turned to the bottom-right quadrant (low-cost, easy to replicate, universal applications) and named the baby sling as an example—any large piece of cloth that can be ingeniously fastened around your body to safely carry a baby. Inventions in this quadrant are cheap, easy to make, and helpful to large groups of people.

Finally, I turned to the bottom-left quadrant (low-cost, highly individualized devices) and explained that this is where I've spent most of my career, with people who trade ideas peer-to-peer about how to create, for example, a way for someone with low dexterity to use a pencil or a workaround for when an alarm on a medical device is too quiet for a deep sleeper.

I paused to take a breath and steal a glance at Dr. Califf, who was listening intently but with no discernible expression on his face. I kept going. I talked about how the ideas that bubble up among patients and caregivers in the lower-left quadrant could be adapted and applied to inventions in the other three quadrants. The internet helps vault people, virtually, out of their home workshops, transporting them into a global conversation about how to improve medical and assistive devices. New capabilities in design, manufacturing, and crowdfunding are allowing new entrants to thrive and experiment at scale. Ideas that were once trapped in inventors' notebooks can now be shared with a worldwide community, tweaked, and then 3D printed in just days. I went on to talk about how we in government could lower the barriers to entry to make it easier for inventors to get access to the resources they need to navigate—for example, the FDA approval process or gain access to a human engineering lab.

Dr. Califf had stayed quiet throughout my presentation, and I worried that I had failed, that I hadn't shown him what was possible. On the contrary. He looked at my drawing and then at me, and said, "In all the years I have spent in health care, I have never considered anything other than the top right quadrant." The other three quadrants had been invisible to him, as he focused exclusively on high-tech device innovation. All of a sudden he could see it: the pent-up energy of all the entrepreneurs and innovators outside the traditional medical and assistive device development pipeline. Previously invisible solutions that people create on their own could become blockbuster products.

Channel this spirit of discovery and possibility. Find and expose blind spots in your organization or industry sector.

CHAMPIONS NEED SEEKERS, NETWORKERS, AND SOLVERS

Too many executives are unaware that the patient-led revolution is churning out improvements and rivals to their services, devices, and treatments. Important innovations are generated by users, every day, beyond the view of corporate research and development labs. That disconnect is costly and not limited to health care.

Researchers in Austria and Germany tallied the most disruptive innovations developed worldwide between 1828 and 2010. They then polled 1,500 executives, clinicians, policymakers, and business professors to see whether these decision-makers could correctly estimate the proportion of user-generated innovations in financial services, medicine, and sport. Only 8 out of 1,500 were able to do so. On average, decision-makers estimated that users came up with just over 21 percent of the most important innovations. The true percentage is 54 percent.[8]

Ignore these numbers at your peril. We need everyone with resources—industry leaders, manufacturers, payers, hospitals, regulators, philanthropists—to recognize that they are at a competitive disadvantage if they are not tapping into rebel health innovation.

Champions: add patients, survivors, and caregivers to your team as evaluators of grants, products, research protocols, and investments. Make sure Seekers, Networkers, and Solvers know how to find you—and, more importantly, how to contribute to your objectives.

CHAMPIONS NEED TO APPOINT AN AMBASSADOR

Jump-start engagement with outside innovators by hiring an ambassador to the Seekers, Networkers, and Solvers who are aligned with your organizational mission. Empower the ambassador with resources, both financial and political (meaning: give them direct access to decision-makers). Make sure both outsiders and insiders, like frontline workers, know that their ideas are welcome.

For example, the Office of the Chief Technology Officer (CTO) at HHS functioned as a one-stop innovation shop for agency leaders and employees who wanted change but were not sure how to pursue it. My predecessors as HHS CTO—Todd Park, who originated the role, and Bryan Sivak, who expanded it—set up agency-wide innovation training programs and gave employees the opportunity to compete for investment in their ideas. The Office of the CTO also recruited people with special talents or work experience outside the federal government to sign up for a one- or two-year tour of duty to solve a particular challenge as an entrepreneur in residence.

These programs helped bring fresh thinking to improve school readiness among low-income children, reduce wait times at Whiteriver Indian Hospital in Arizona, ensure the safety of the organ donation tracking system, and create an open-source library of 3D-printable biomedical models at NIH, to name just four projects. If not for the Office of the CTO and the sponsorship of the HHS leadership, none of these innovations would have been able to survive the usual bureaucratic process and strict hierarchy of a federal agency.

An ambassador can also come from outside your organization, such as Howard Look of Tidepool or Jen Horonjeff of Savvy Cooperative. They are able to recruit Seekers, Networkers, and Solvers to join a cause that aligns with both their mission and a company's bottom line.

CHAMPIONS NEED TO HOLD PRIZE COMPETITIONS

Sometimes a problem was so complex that HHS leaders were not sure what kind of expertise they needed. They wanted out-of-the-box ideas from all kinds of people. That's when we would recommend a prize competition.

Prize competitions (also called challenges) have been used since the eighteenth century by both public and private-sector organizations to spark innovation and recruit people to a cause. Napoleon's government, for example, sponsored a prize competition to find a new way to preserve food for an army on the move. (The winner, Nicolas François Appert, essentially invented canning.) More recently, NASA awarded three prizes to outside innovators who came up with new methods to measure the strain capacity of Kevlar and Vectran straps in a wide range of temperatures. One of the three winners has no formal training in materials science.

To give you an idea of the scope of the field, the US government has sponsored over 1,200 prize competitions since the passage of the America COMPETES Reauthorization Act of 2010. InnoCentive, a company that runs prize competitions, has a worldwide network of over 500,000 problem-solvers and has fostered the creation of more than 200,000 new products and services since its founding in 1998.

Prizes can be either monetary or symbolic, like a medal. And since they are designed to be open, anyone with a great idea can win.

Indeed, one finalist for an HHS prize competition was a high school student. Because he was younger than the required minimum age of eighteen, David Li used his father's name to enter his idea for tracking durable medical equipment during natural disasters. He came in third place, and he used his prize money to further develop his device, which he later brought to Washington, DC, to share with HHS leaders. (He also summarized his work in a paper for high school class credit.) Li is an example of a Solver whose drive to contribute was so strong that he jumped over every obstacle in his path.

Prize competitions are an intake valve for fresh thinking and a pathway for executives to become Champions. The exercise of clearly and publicly describing a problem is useful in itself since it demands honesty and transparency. Listen and learn from the Solvers who compete, then spotlight and support the best solutions.

CHAMPIONS NEED TO CONNECT SOLVERS WITH EXPERTS AND FUNDING

One of the challenges that Solvers face is not having access to the expertise they need to perfect the product they are creating. A Champion can help bridge that gap.

When the FDA launched its first prize competition—the Food Safety Challenge—it called on academic institutions and industry laboratories to develop new ways to detect salmonella in fresh produce. The agency's audacious goal was to cut detection time from five days to five hours.

Five finalists were awarded $20,000 to develop their ideas. Finalists also received expert advice from an FDA mentor—a customer or future user of the product, in private-sector terms.

As the executive sponsor for the competition, I attended the showcase at the close of the challenge and saw how a relatively minor investment had already yielded a range of excellent new ideas to improve food safety. Remarkably, all five team leaders told me that, while they hoped to win, the $300,000 grand prize purse was secondary to the opportunity to work with an FDA mentor, a customer for the kind of work they do in their labs. They said they are otherwise barred from communicating with the FDA because of the strict regulations separating regulators from anyone who might influence their important work, safeguarding the nation's food supply.

No surprise, when I asked my colleagues at the FDA, they told me they deeply appreciated the chance to talk with the designers of the solutions. To tell them, for example, "That device won't fit in the back of my car. You have to make it smaller." Or, "This device has to be more durable. It's going to get knocked around as we take it from site to site."

The prize competition was a pop-up community of practice, a temporary space where customers (FDA employees) and Solvers (device designers) could exchange ideas and collaborate. In this scenario, the agency's leaders acted as Champions, connecting the two groups by sponsoring the prize competition. And although the Solvers were not patient-led, the lessons hold.

The winning team, from Purdue University, used part of the prize money to fund undergraduate and graduate students' research and training, further expanding the field of people who can contribute to the ongoing work of food safety. This was a multilevel win: the FDA got specific, new technology, and the field got reinvigorated more generally.

If you want to encourage change in a certain sector of the health-care industry, consider how you might set up a competition that results in unrestricted funds going to the winning teams. Solvers will know how to deploy those resources.

CHAMPIONS NEED TO PRIORITIZE PATIENT-LED TEAMS

In 2018, HHS partnered with the American Society of Nephrology to spark innovation in the prevention and treatment of kidney diseases. The resulting initiative—KidneyX—fielded a series of prize competitions to redesign dialysis, accelerate artificial kidney development, and improve patients' quality of life.

KidneyX has consistently sought to include grassroots, patient-led teams, such as when they focused on how to reduce the transmission of coronavirus in clinical settings. As the three sponsors of the initiative wrote, "By designing this prize challenge to directly solicit solutions from people at the ground level, we not only involved them in the research process, we gained better understanding of challenges that are being faced in everyday care centers."[9] KidneyX joins two strong forces: open innovation, which invites participation from a broad population with diverse skill sets, and patient-led innovation, which requires deep, specific experiences with the problems being solved.

Winnie Cheng, a kidney disease patient, led one of the winning teams responding to the challenges of the pandemic. She worried about how vulnerable people like herself would be able to get access to healthy foods when the virus was rampant and immune-compromised people were told to stay home. She came up with an idea for a home-delivery service of renal-friendly foods and asked her online patient community for feedback. Other kidney disease patients enthusiastically endorsed the idea of StockMyPantry, writing that they were afraid to go out shopping or were unable to leave the house at all. Another wrote, "Not only do people need help with food, they need to be reminded they aren't forgotten."

Cheng built a GoFundMe page that raised more than $13,000 and made over two hundred deliveries in thirty-eight states. KidneyX provided funding to continue the work and something less tangible, but no less important: a reputation boost. Cheng has expanded StockMyPantry's capacity for patient education about the importance of following a healthy diet.

By sponsoring prize competitions that specifically recruited Networker-Solvers, the KidneyX sponsors became Champions, helping people like Cheng to serve her fellow patients.

CHAMPIONS NEED TO FIND NETWORKER-SOLVERS

Networkers play a crucial role at every stage of the entrepreneurial process, from ideation to commercialization and diffusion. Christoph Hienerth and Christopher Lettl, the innovation researchers I mentioned in chapter 8, documented case studies of eight innovators in two very different fields: surgical tools and kayaking gear. They looked at patterns of success and failure across the life cycle of a new piece of medical or sporting equipment and their findings light a path for patient-led innovators to follow.

In all eight case studies, innovators sought out and listened to the people in their fields who said they were dissatisfied with existing techniques and equipment. In the rebel health model, that is the equivalent of Solvers and Champions reaching out to Seekers and Networkers who identify and publicize gaps in the market.

Innovators then shared early concepts for improvements or new devices with peers, whether they were surgeons or elite kayakers, and collected feedback. Again, this is like when members of the diabetes rebel alliance shared their prototypes of Nightscout or OpenAPS with fellow patients and caregivers to improve the code or design.

Here's a key insight: Incumbent organizations with a comfortable market share, who seek to please a majority of users, are more likely to collect information about the *average* user. Innovators, meanwhile, collect information about *lead* users. That explains why established device manufacturers did not see the patient-led revolution coming—they were not paying attention to the conversations happening among Seekers, Networkers, and Solvers.

Hienerth and Lettl observe that those who invest in peer relationships are more likely to get the conceptual advice they need on their innovations. Champions should look for Solvers who are also Networkers since people who are well-known in their community will be more likely to get that useful feedback. Solvers who work alone are likely to be slowed down by a lack of input. The only exceptions are superstars, like a world champion kayaker or a surgeon who leads their field, whose fame can draw people to their cause.

CHAMPIONS NEED TO HELP SOLVERS SCALE

Solvers' needs shift in later-stage product development. Access to money, materials, data, and labs is essential. This is when Champions shine. They can monitor lead-user communities and spot emerging opportunities for new products and services. If they see a team of Solvers that has created something of value for their peers, Champions can provide the support they need to scale it up for a wider audience, as Abbott did when it invested in Bigfoot Biomedical and its smart insulin pen or when Roche acquired mySugr (figure 10.2).

Solvers can try to get Champions' attention by presenting at high-profile industry events or entering and winning competitions. Networkers can help Solvers amplify their messages at this stage, spreading the word about their accomplishments to a wider audience.

Champions who cultivate connections with Seekers, Networkers, and Solvers are more likely to be able to spot opportunities in their field. And an innovation is more likely to reach a majority of potential users and become the new standard when it is supported by both a community of Networkers and the resources a Champion can provide.[10]

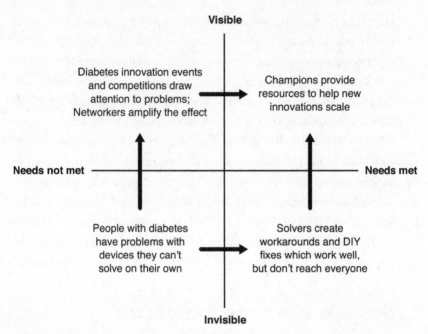

Figure 10.2
Rebel Health Matrix: Diabetes.

CHAMPIONS NEED TO HELP REBELS BRIDGE THE CREDIBILITY GAP

Rebels move quickly to identify and solve problems that are not yet visible to mainstream institutions. But they often have a credibility gap, which prevents their discoveries from reaching everyone who could benefit from them, from fellow patients who face the same challenges to researchers with generous funding and world-class labs. The result is that too many great patient- and community-generated ideas die in obscurity.

One solution is to help outside innovators gain credibility through academic publication.

For example, Dana Lewis was first a Networker, building her reputation as the leader of an online community of health-care innovators by running the Healthcare Communications & Social Media community (#hcsm) on Twitter for nine years. She then emerged as a diabetes device Solver and built up her academic and industry credentials by presenting at scientific meetings and publishing journal articles and a book about open-source diabetes solutions. The Robert Wood Johnson Foundation, the largest public health philanthropic organization in the United States and a Champion for pioneering, patient-led innovation, recognized Lewis's leadership and funded her research.

Lewis is both a medical device hacker and a bureaucracy hacker. She meticulously documented the barriers she encountered on her way to gaining credibility and then built tools to open pathways for other citizen-scientists. By highlighting the challenges of data collection and analysis, as well as real and perceived requirements of participation in academic conferences and publication, Lewis drew a map for Champions who want to help rebels navigate these unfamiliar waters.[11] An established organization can build a track record of respectful collaboration with patients, mentoring those who seek publication or a conference speaker slot. Lewis also recommends taking advantage of the media spotlight, as Long COVID patients did in 2020, leveraging the attention to further their cause of patient-led research. Champions can assist by asking patients to appear with them on conference panels or making sure that any reporter who calls them for a quote also has the contact information for patients, survivors, and caregivers who can provide insights.

CHAMPIONS NEED TO OPEN DOORS

Lisa D. Cook, an economist and member of the Federal Reserve Board of Governors, has documented how women and underrepresented minorities have been discriminated against at every stage of the innovation process. As she writes, "This innovation gap represents a lost opportunity, a discriminatory drag on our economy, and further structural evidence of the wide income and wealth gaps in the United States."[12]

Champions of patient-led health innovation can learn from Cook and her colleagues about how to create opportunities for everyone to participate. Equal access to education and training is key, as is making sure that the doors to labs and workshops are open to everyone who has ideas to contribute. Senior-level expertise and experience are additional resources to be shared by Champions. Mentors can guide a Solver's work, make connections with funders, and convince other institutions to help.

For example, the FDA Food Safety Challenge paired outside innovators with inside experts, creating a temporary mentorship program that helped new ideas flourish. In this way, FDA leaders were Champions for both their own food inspectors, whose need for better tools was not visible to innovators, and for Solvers in the private sector, who would otherwise not have access to the resources they need to develop their concepts (figure 10.3).

As we saw in chapter 3, Don Berwick, MD, invited Sorrel King to be part of the group working on a patient safety campaign, giving her access to an audience full of clinicians who were ready to hear her message about a caregiver-led response to medical errors. Berwick acted as a Champion, highlighting the previously unseen infrastructure of family members who could act as early warning systems at the bedside (figure 10.4).

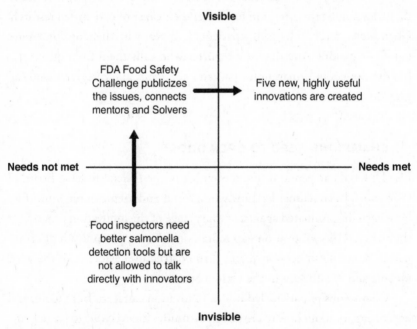

Figure 10.3
Rebel Health Matrix: Food safety.

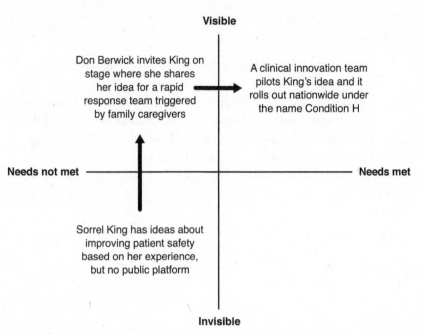

Visible

Don Berwick invites King on stage where she shares her idea for a rapid response team triggered by family caregivers

A clinical innovation team pilots King's idea and it rolls out nationwide under the name Condition H

Needs not met —————————————————— Needs met

Sorrel King has ideas about improving patient safety based on her experience, but no public platform

Invisible

Figure 10.4
Rebel Health Matrix: Patient safety.

In a similar vein, the NBCC trains laypeople to take their seats at the research table along with scientists and clinicians, as do other patient-led organizations like the Tigerlily Foundation and GRASP Cancer (Guiding Researchers and Advocates to Scientific Partnerships). These Champion organizations prepare patients, survivors, and caregivers to contribute to the high-level discussions, winning the respect that they deserve but do not always receive. Needs not met become visible to mainstream institutions that are open to input from these new sources, enabling resources to flow to the most pressing problems.

Takeaways:

1. Champions need to help Solvers break new paths through the permafrost of the status quo.
2. Champions spotlight and support the best solutions, even when they come from unusual sources because they know that blind spots are costly.
3. Champions find ways to build teams of Solvers from inside their organizations or open doors to outside innovators.

11 GET STARTED

My passion for the patient-led revolution is both professional and personal.

I grew up rich in cousins. I spent holidays with my first cousins and lived, starting at age eleven, in the same town with second cousins (the children of my mother's first cousin) and a first cousin twice removed (my grandmother's first cousin—each generation that separates us is the "removed" part). Don't worry, there won't be a quiz.

As the third child of three in my own family and in the middle of the pack, age-wise, among all my cousins, I often longed for special attention from elders. I found it in my relationship with my grandmother's first cousin and her husband, Ann and Mitsuru Yasuhara. They were mathematicians who delighted in logic games, musicians with strong opinions about composers and performances, and as elegant and worldly as my middle-school brain could imagine. They had no children.

Mitsuru grew up in Japan during World War II and came to the United States for graduate school. Ann grew up in Wisconsin. They met at a party in Illinois and got married—a bold act for the 1960s, a Japanese man marrying a White woman.

The first time I visited their home in Princeton, New Jersey, we sat on pillows around a low table, Japanese style. I was so inexperienced and eager at age eleven that I added both milk and lemon to my tea, curdling it. Ann endeared herself to me forever with her gentle smile and quick explanation of the science experiment I'd accidentally conducted.

There are many more stories to tell since that day over forty years ago, but I'll fast-forward to the moment when Mitsuru asked me to be his caregiver.

Ann had died a few years before, leaving him alone in their snug home filled with books, records, and art. Mitsuru did not like change of any sort, and Ann's death was the most unwelcome change imaginable.

With a deep bow of honor, I accepted. I had helped care for my father for the year before he died and, as I told Mitsuru, I entered into this new caregiving relationship with my eyes open, knowing the length, depth, and breadth of what he was asking of me. I said yes to it all.

I think I saw his shoulders drop about an inch when I accepted. In that moment, I felt all the belonging, all the love that had been stored up in me by Ann and Mitsuru come rushing forward. What do we want to do in life but be there, in those moments, in fellowship with another human? What higher use is there for my time and energy?

Because I am a Networker, I had prepared for this conversation by pooling resources gleaned from peer caregivers. I selected tools to help us jump up a few levels in our relationship, to transform ourselves from fond friends to trusted partners.

The first topic I introduced was the end of life. I wanted to plunge into a conversation about death as a symbol of how serious we both were about this new stage of our shared journey. I needed to know what he wanted so I could fight for it, if need be.

I chose Engage with Grace, a tool developed by Alexandra Drane, a Solver and Champion who cofounded Archangels, a company that lifts up caregivers. Mitsuru was neutral on the question of dying at home versus in a hospital, but he had a definite opinion about interventions ("palliative care, yes; resurrection, no"). Happily, he was in good health, so this was not an urgent conversation. He regularly bicycled to the grocery store and to Quaker meetings, hosted dinner parties, and attended the opera in New York City.

Turning to the CareMap tool developed by Rajiv Mehta, another Solver-Champion who runs the nonprofit Atlas of Care, Mitsuru and I were able to assemble a list of neighbors, friends, vendors, and clinicians he relies on. After I drove back home to Washington, DC, that day, Mitsuru called the inner circle of his support network to let them know that they were part of his CareMap. Some of them told me later that they were deeply touched to hear this, and I realized that a byproduct of the CareMap is a rippling wave of love, from the center and then back again as they accepted their roles on Mitsuru's team.

As a practical matter, getting all those phone numbers in one place was very helpful when Mitsuru got sick two years later. Thanks to the CareMap, I was able to organize food delivery and visits from local friends, even under pandemic restrictions. Thanks to Engage with Grace, I had Mitsuru's end-of-life wishes documented and organized, which gave me both the courage and the authority as his health-care proxy to stop the machinery of fruitless treatment. I'll never forget his smile as I stood in his hospital room doorway and said no to that last blood draw. We were able to navigate our way out of the health care system when his diagnosis was terminal and codesign a home hospice that honored his wishes for a peaceful death. He died at home, with birds singing in the garden as I wafted steam from a cup of his favorite tea toward his final breaths.

My success as a caregiver was due to the work I put in as Networker, constantly gathering resources to share with Mitsuru.

I'm sharing this story not to brag about what a great Networker I am but to set the scene for the following confession: the first time I faced a health crisis in my family, I failed. I had been tracking the patient-led revolution for a few years, gathering evidence of how useful it is for patients, survivors, and caregivers to seek answers, pool resources, and solve problems together. But I did not think that I needed to tap into that vein of wisdom and innovation for myself.

Maybe you are like me. You think you've got it all together in terms of your health. When you have a question, you Google it, and the information you need generally pops up. If you're lucky, you already have a doctor you trust and friends who pitch in with practical advice and emotional support.

It's easy to assume you have the best available knowledge. I did. When my younger child was diagnosed with life-threatening food allergies I thought we could handle it on our own as a family. I read a few articles online. I bought a couple of books. I found an allergist. I thought I had it all together

I was wrong.

I didn't know that one of the world's foremost experts in food allergy practiced just an hour away and was taking new patients. I didn't know that the local clinical practice we had chosen was using outdated testing procedures. I didn't know that we had to change how we shopped, stored, and cooked food, both at home and when traveling. I didn't know that there are restaurants that cater to people with food allergies. I didn't know any of the local or federal regulations around carrying epinephrine, which can stop a reaction if used immediately. Heck, I didn't even fill the prescription for an epinephrine auto-injector until after our second trip to the emergency room.

My confident Google searches brought none of those revelations. No, the epiphany came offline, when my husband's colleague Julia Gordon invited us to join her online community of Washington, DC-area food allergy families. I had assumed that support groups were for other, more desperate people, not me. I did not think I had anything to learn from fellow parents.

Tapping into peer knowledge meant we were able to ask for more precise tests, get into a clinical trial, and cut in half the list of foods to avoid. It also taught me how to be a Networker. Thanks to the lessons learned from my experience as a food allergy advocate, I could be a more effective caregiver for other people in my life, like Mitsuru.

My goal in writing this book has been to help you see what I see: the wide horizon and abundant opportunities presented by an underground revolution in health and health care. I hope you take inspiration from the ways that Seekers, Networkers, Solvers, and Champions have navigated the health-care maze faster than other people. You can make a difference for yourself, for the people you love, and for the organizations you lead.

When a crisis hits, you can recognize patterns and say, "OK, I need to become a Seeker and go out on the hunt," or "Let's look for Networkers and Solvers whose skill sets can help us." Sometimes a health challenge calls for support and circling in. Sometimes it calls for change and reaching out.

There are two ways to apply these ideas:

1) To help one person (yourself or someone else)
2) To help a group (members of a health plan, for example, patients in a hospital system, people who share the same condition, or residents of a region or country)

Either way, the first step is to figure out where you are on the Rebel Health Matrix.

FIND YOURSELF

How would you characterize the challenge you face? Is the problem mysterious and therefore not yet visible to most people? Is there a solution that has not yet spread to everyone who could benefit? Or is it a known and visible concern, but people's needs are not being met? Here's the playbook for each quadrant (figures 11.1–11.4).

SCENARIO #1: NEEDS NOT MET, INVISIBLE TO MAINSTREAM HEALTH CARE

If the challenges you face are in the lower-left quadrant, you need to become or recruit a Seeker. A Seeker will go and find out if there are useful resources currently hidden from view. Remember how Brett Alder searched online for fellow sufferers in chapter 2 and Kyra Hagan managed to stumble on a

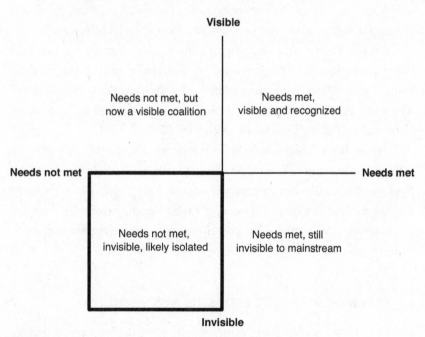

Figure 11.1
Rebel Health Matrix: Needs not met, invisible to mainstream health care.

just-in-time someone-like-her in chapter 3? They borrowed tactics and courage to climb out of their predicaments and into the upper-right quadrant, where a solution was at hand.

You also need to become or recruit a Networker like the ones I profiled in chapters 4 and 5. Draw inspiration from Vicki McCarrell, who helped build the Moebius Syndrome Foundation, or Fiona Lowenstein, whose online organizing and *New York Times* essays shone a light on the emerging population of people living with Long COVID. Networkers can raise the visibility of a challenge and bring together teams of people who may otherwise never know each other. Together, Seekers and Networkers can hunt and gather, defining and prioritizing the problems that need to be solved.

The next step is to invite Solvers into the conversation. You can do this by publicizing your frustration, as we saw in chapter 8 when Jimmy Choi posted a TikTok video excoriating pharmaceutical companies for making pills so small. Brian Alldridge and his Solver collaborators answered the call. A hashtag like the diabetes community's #WeAreNotWaiting can be a beacon for Solvers who want to contribute their skills (see chapter 9).

You can also attract Solvers by holding a prize competition. Look for ways to make it easy for anyone to quickly understand and dig into the challenge you face. Solvers may come forward with ideas that you may never have come up with on your own, as the organizers of the FDA Food Safety Challenge or KidneyX found out in chapter 10.

Remember to look for ways to get Solvers what they need, such as access to the tools, information, and data that are essential for tackling a challenge. Find out who is blocking access and borrow Amy Tenderich's strategy of inviting them to join your next meeting. Or find an ambassador like Howard Look, someone who can broker a détente among competing interests (both stories from chapter 9).

SCENARIO #2: NEEDS MET, STILL NOT VISIBLE

If the challenge you face is in the lower-right quadrant—people's needs are being met, but only a few people know about the solution or tool—then it is time to either become or recruit a Networker to raise its visibility or a

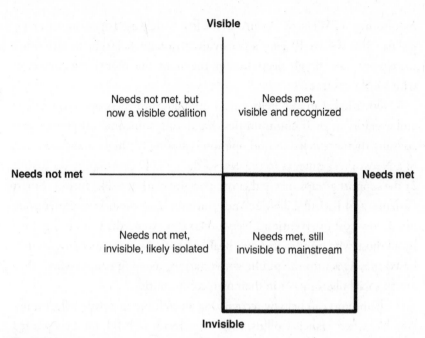

Figure 11.2

Rebel Health Matrix: Needs met, still invisible.

Champion who can provide the resources necessary to scale up a peer-led idea.

Effective Networkers can help make sure that everyone who could benefit from an innovation is able to understand it, get it, and, if necessary, keep at it. Networkers can say to people who share their condition or life stage, "This works! I use it myself." They can leverage the authority of lived experience to help someone else adopt a new behavior or device. Without that support, people often give up. Innovations and proven treatments don't spread and take hold for the long term.

The DOC is a sentinel example of Networkers who educate people who are newly diagnosed or newly committed to better health. From everyday advice about meal planning to in-depth coaching to get a newly diagnosed patient set up for success, Networkers in the DOC spread the word about innovations and strategies. On Facebook, people teach each other how to set up their own rigs, whether for Nightscout, the rogue workaround for remote monitoring of PWDs, or OpenAPS, the first widely used open-source artificial pancreas system. Patients and caregivers donate their time to each other to help one more family sleep through the night, one more kid go to school with a little less fear.

Networkers can also help spread public health messages and work as ambassadors in their communities. Validating someone's suspicions and advising them to seek a second opinion is among the highest and best uses of a Networker's time, as in the case of the /r/STD community on Reddit or the support groups that gather on specialty platforms like Inspire, Smart Patients, and PatientsLikeMe. And, since some of the best treatments are no- or low-cost interventions, Networkers can extend the work being done by all those who want to improve health-care delivery by injecting science-based messages into the public conversation, meeting people where they are on social platforms or in their own communities.

Champions can help by recognizing and lifting up a patient-led initiative, like when Francis Collins, then the director of NIH, publicly praised the work of the Patient-Led Research Collaborative's Long COVID studies. Or when Genentech partnered with the NBCC to speed clinical trial recruitment, knowing that they could not reach their goals without those skilled patient- and survivor-led organizers, as we saw in chapter 10. We make real progress when Champions follow up with funding and other support beyond media attention or a one-time collaboration.

SCENARIO #3: NEEDS NOT MET, VISIBLE

If the challenge you face is well-known, but nobody has solved it yet, you need to recruit or become a Solver or a Champion.

The #WeAreNotWaiting movement was born out of the frustration of people living with diabetes being told to be patient while scientists and health-care leaders worked on it. Solvers emerged from within the diabetes community. They created Nightscout, OpenAPS, smart insulin pens, and other patient-led innovations. The rebel alliance threw a spotlight on what PWDs and their loved ones needed. Eventually, the federal government

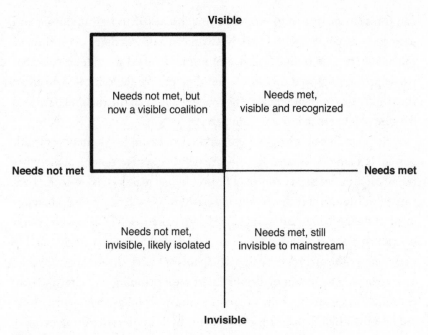

Figure 11.3
Rebel Health Matrix: Needs not met, now visible.

and savvy industry leaders took notes and supported the DOC's call for change.

The US health-care system is shifting toward value-based care, meaning hospitals and clinicians are paid based on patients' health outcomes (the value of the care) instead of on the number of procedures performed (the volume of care). Everyone benefits when people avoid complications and stay well. This points to the economic case for tapping into peer expertise to meet the needs of people who face well-understood challenges. It is an opportunity for Champions to step forward.

As we saw in chapter 4, peer-to-peer patient and survivor networks aid in the management of a wide range of chronic conditions, including some of the most expensive and complicated populations to treat, such as organ transplant recipients and people with insulin-requiring diabetes. Medication adherence is a perennial issue for every age and disease group. Champions can invest in platforms to attract people interested in learning more and help them become Seekers and Networkers. For example, two-thirds of the members of an online health community focused on epilepsy said that participation improved their understanding of how their disease will affect them and one-third said they are now better about taking their medications because of what they learned from peers.[1]

Help can come both online and offline. For example, Montefiore Health System is a large integrated health-care delivery system serving a safety net population in the Bronx and the Hudson Valley region of New York. They turned to InquisitHealth, a company based in New Jersey, to help manage some of their toughest cases. InquisitHealth paired each person with poorly controlled diabetes with a mentor based on shared culture, language, and life experiences. The mentors visited participants at home, checked in by phone, or used an app to answer questions about meal planning, exercise, and care coordination. A study of the program found that, on average, participants reduced their blood glucose measurements by 1.7 points, resulting in fewer complications and lower costs.[2]

By hiring InquisitHealth, Montefiore's leaders became Champions of an innovation powered by patients, survivors, and caregivers. Participating patients are more likely to stay well and enjoy the benefits of being in the top right quadrant of the Rebel Health Matrix, where their challenges are visible and their needs are met.

SCENARIO #4: NEEDS MET, VISIBLE AND RECOGNIZED

If you and the people you love or serve are in the upper-right quadrant, you are dealing with problems that are visible to mainstream health care and there are known cures, good therapies, and useful devices. The issue may be a temporary condition, like a broken arm or healthy pregnancy. Challenges experienced by people in this quadrant are likely to be related to access to solutions and the cost of care. A drug or device may be out of reach because a clinician won't prescribe it or insurance won't cover it. Or a surgeon who can perform a certain procedure is not available in your region. These challenges fall outside the scope of this book but are another frontier of the patient-led revolution.

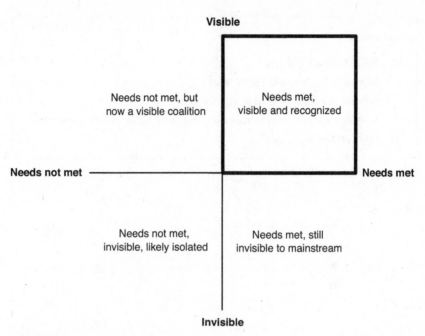

Visible

Needs not met, but
now a visible coalition

Needs met,
visible and recognized

Needs not met —————————————— **Needs met**

Needs not met,
invisible, likely isolated

Needs met, still
invisible to mainstream

Invisible

Figure 11.4
Rebel Health Matrix: Needs met, visible to mainstream health care.

CONCLUSION

If you are a Seeker, keep going—the answers are out there. If you are a Networker, continue pooling resources and sharing the best of what you and your community can find. If you are a Solver, start building what you think should exist. If you are a Champion, look for ways to open doors to rebels.

There are Seekers, Networkers, Solvers, and Champions all over the world working toward system transformation. I maintain a list of organizations and companies that are leveraging patient-led innovation on my website: https://susannahfox.com/patient-led-innovation/. If you have influence, invest in them, partner with them, and find ways to boost their signal within your own communities. If you are waiting for a sign that it's time to change the way you approach health and health care, then this is it. Join the revolution!

Takeaways:

1. Seekers: Don't give up.
2. Networkers: Spread the good stuff.
3. Solvers: Start building what you think should exist.
4. Champions: Create opportunities for teams led by patients, survivors, and caregivers.

Acknowledgments

The patient-led revolution is playing out on social platforms and I am indebted to the patients, survivors, and caregivers who share their stories, openly and bravely. You light the way for all of us.

To the Seekers, Networkers, Solvers, and Champions who shared their wisdom, thank you: Natalie Abbott; Brett Alder; Brian Alldridge; Gina Assaf; Deanna Attai, MD; Anat Bar-Cohen; Stayce Beck, PhD; Jan Berger, MD; Tracy Behrsing; Amrita Bhowmick; Kathleen Bogart, PhD; John Bostick; Diane Breton; Jeffrey Brewer; Helen Burstin, MD; Robert Califf, MD; Hugo Campos; Winnie Cheng, PhD; Larry Chu, MD; Hannah Davis; LaTonya Davis; Maris Degenere; Lane Desborough; Ellen Di Resta; Andrea Downing; Amanda Dykeman; Hannah Eichner; Javier Evelyn; David Fajgenbaum, MD; Lisa Fitzpatrick, MD; Billie Friedman; Lotus Friedman; Gilles Frydman; Jose Gomez-Marquez; Kyra Hagan; Rose Hedges, DNP RN; Ben Heywood; Jamie Heywood; Jill Holdren; Sara Holoubek; Jen Horonjeff, PhD; Matthew Joffe; Carmen Kleinsmith, MSN, RN; David Kozin; Emily Kramer-Golinkoff; Gokul Krishnan; Harlan Krumholz, MD; Bon Ku, MD; Michael R. Ladisch, PhD; Jack Lennon; Dana Lewis; Stephanie Lieber; Doug Lindsay; Craig Lipset; Michelle Litchman, PhD, FNP; Brian Loew; Howard Look; Fiona Lowenstein; Barbara Lubash; Wendy Lynch, PhD; Peter Margolis, MD; Kedar Mate, MD; Julia Maués; Katie McCurdy; Bryan Mazlish; Vicki McCarrell; Anna McCollister; Delina Pryce McPhaull; Rajiv Mehta; Matt Might, PhD; Nell Minow; Erin Moore; Hil Moss; Sally Okun, RN; JD Ouellette; Corrie Painter, PhD; Erin Parks, PhD; Ashwin Patel,

MD; Sandeep Patel, PhD; Ryan Prior; Vincent Rajkumar, MD; Howard Rheingold; Vicky Rideout; Sara Riggare, PhD; Camila Ronderos, PhD; Seth Rotberg; Kristina Saffran; Sean Saint; Liz Salmi; Susan Schaffler; Michael Seid, PhD; Carolyn Wong Simpkins, MD; Christopher Snider; Paul Tarini; Amy Tenderich; Solome Tibebu; Carissa Tozzi; Gayle Vaday; Fran Visco; Eric von Hippel, PhD; Ben West; Paul Wicks, PhD; Louise Wides; Anna Young; Colleen Young; Matthew Zachary; George Zamanakos, PhD.

I gained insights on the patient-led scientific revolution from the following authors and their work: Steven Epstein, *Impure Science*; Dana M. Lewis, *Automated Insulin Delivery*; Fiona Lowenstein, editor, *The Long COVID Survival Guide*; Amy Dockser Marcus, *We the Scientists*; Alondra Nelson, *Body and Soul*; Ryan Prior, *The Long Haul*; Sara Riggare, *Personal Science in Parkinson's Disease*.

These authors expanded my perspective on the patient and caregiver experience: Susannah Cahalan, *Brain on Fire*; e-Patient Dave deBronkart, *Laugh, Sing, and Eat Like a Pig*; Ross Douthat, *The Deep Places*; Sorrel King, *Josie's Story*; Susannah Meadows, *The Other Side of Impossible*; Abby Norman, *Ask Me About My Uterus*; Meghan O'Rourke, *The Invisible Kingdom*; Siren Interactive, *Uncommon Challenges; Shared Journeys*; Laurie Strongin, *Saving Henry*; Mary Elizabeth Williams, *A Series of Catastrophes and Miracles*.

The following authors deepened my understanding of health care: Paul Batalden, editor, *Lessons Learned in Changing Healthcare and How We Learned Them*; Robert Bazell, *HER-2*; Jan Berger and Julie Slezak, *Reengaging in Trust*; e-Patient Dave deBronkart with Danny Sands, MD, *Let Patients Help*; David Fajgenbaum, MD, *Chasing My Cure*; Tom Ferguson, MD, *Medical Self-Care; Health Online; e-Patients*; Diana E. Forsythe, *Studying Those Who Study Us*; Jan Oldenburg, editor, *Engage!*; Victor Montori, MD, *Why We Revolt*.

Bob Prior, an executive editor at MIT Press, shared my vision for this book from our very first conversation and created space for me to build it. Thanks also to Jessica Pellien for her guidance and encouragement.

My sister, Elizabeth Fox, is my thought partner, most spirited cheerleader, and toughest critic, as only a sibling can be.

Thank you to my early draft readers: Dave deBronkart; Abbe Don; Barbara Figge Fox; Mark Ganz; Felicia M.T. Lewis, MD; Christopher Schroeder; Gary Wolf. I would also like to thank the MIT Press anonymous reviewers for their comments and questions. Special thanks to Barbara Spindel for running the final lap with me.

I am grateful to Roni Ayalla and Michael Bean for designing the illustrations and to Clara Ganz for the cover concept.

A toast to my peer mentors, whose insights and enthusiasm spurred me on: Alexandra Drane; Jodi Ferrier, Margaret Laws; Jane Sarasohn-Kahn; Laurie Strongin; Lisa Suennen, Paige Trevor; Wendy Sue Swanson, MD; Matthew Trowbridge, MD; Roni Zeiger, MD.

Thank you to my parents, George and Barbara Fox, and my in-laws, Dan and Marcia Halperin, for your support and love.

Most of all, thank you Eric, Scarlette, and Rain, loves of my life.

Notes

CHAPTER 1

1. Alondra Nelson, "Spin Doctors: The Politics of Sickle Cell Anemia," in *Body and Soul: The Black Panther Party and the Fight Against Medical Discrimination* (Minneapolis: University of Minnesota Press, 2013), 115–52.

2. Mary T. Bassett, "No Justice, No Health: The Black Panther Party's Fight for Health in Boston and Beyond," *Journal of African American Studies* 23 (November 2019): 352–63, https://doi .org/10.1007/s12111-019-09450-w.

3. Alfredo Morabia, "Unveiling the Black Panther Party Legacy to Public Health," *American Journal of Public Health* 106, no. 10 (October 2016): 1732–33, https://doi.org/10.2105 /AJPH.2016.303405.

4. Steven Epstein, *Impure Science: AIDS, Activism, and the Politics of Knowledge* (Berkeley: University of California Press, 1996), 218–219.

5. Christopher Knoepke, D. Hogan Slack, M. Pilar Ingle, Daniel D. Matlock, and Lucas N. Marzec, "Quality of Medical Advice Provided between Members of a Web-Based Message Board for Patients with Implantable Defibrillators: Mixed-Methods Study," *JMIR Cardio* 2, no. 2 (2018), https://doi.org/10.2196/11358.

CHAPTER 2

1. Alicia L. Nobles, Eric C. Leas, Benjamin M. Althouse, Mark Dredze, Christopher A. Longhurst, Davey M. Smith, and John W. Ayers, "Requests for Diagnoses of Sexually Transmitted Diseases on a Social Media Platform," *Journal of the American Medical Association* 322, no. 17 (2019), https://doi.org/10.1001/jama.2019.14390.

2. Marcel D. Waldinger, Marcus M.H.M. Meinardi, Aeilko H. Zwinderman, and Dave H. Schweitzer, "Postorgasmic Illness Syndrome (POIS) in 45 Dutch Caucasian Males: Clinical Characteristics and Evidence for an Immunogenic Pathogenesis (Part 1)," *The Journal of Sexual Medicine* 8, no. 4 (2011), https://doi.org/10.1111/j.1743-6109.2010.02166.x.

3. Diana E. Forsythe, "New Bottles, Old Wine: Hidden Cultural Assumptions in a Computerized Explanation System for Migraine Sufferers," in *Studying Those Who Study Us: An Anthropologist in the World of Artificial Intelligence*, ed. David J. Hess (Redwood City: Stanford University Press, 2002), 93–118.

CHAPTER 3

1. Deborah Tallon, Jiri Chard, and Paul Dieppe, "Relation between Agendas of the Research Community and the Research Consumer," *The Lancet* 355, no. 9220 (June 2000): 2037–2040, https://doi.org/10.1016/S0140-6736(00)02351-5.

2. Katherine H.O. Deane, Helen Flaherty, David J. Daley, Roland Pascoe, Bridget Penhale, Carl E. Clark, Catherine Sackley, and Stacey Storey, "Priority Setting Partnership to Identify the Top 10 Research Priorities for the Management of Parkinson's Disease," *BMJ Open* 4, (2014): e006434, https://doi.org/10.1136/bmjopen-2014-006434.

3. Tom Ferguson, MD, *e-Patients: How They Can Help Us Heal Healthcare*, e-patients.net, 2007. Quoted with permission.

4. Tara Kirk Sell, Divya Hosangadi, Elizabeth Smith, Marc Trotochaud, Prarthana Vasudevan, Gigi Kwik Gronvall, Yonaira Rivera, Jeannette Sutton, Alex Ruiz, and Anita Cicero, *National Priorities to Combat Misinformation and Disinformation for COVID-19 and Future Public Health Threats: A Call for a National Strategy* (Baltimore, MD: Johns Hopkins Center for Health Security; 2021), https://www.centerforhealthsecurity.org/our-work/pubs_archive/pubs-pdfs/2021/210322-misinformation.pdf.

5. Sorrel King, *Josie's Story: A Mother's Inspiring Crusade to Make Medical Care Safe* (New York: Grove Press, 2009), 195–196.

6. Jonathan R. Welch, "As She Lay Dying: How I Fought to Stop Medical Errors from Killing My Mom," *Health Affairs*, December 2012, https://doi/10.1377/hlthaff.2012.0833.

CHAPTER 4

1. Howard Rheingold, *The Virtual Community: Homesteading on the Electronic Frontier* (Cambridge: MIT Press, 1993), https://www.rheingold.com/vc/book/intro.html.

2. Jay Allison, "Vigil," *JayAllison.com* (blog), September 15, 1989, http://jayallison.com/vigil/.

3. Gretchen K. Berland, Marc N. Elliott, Leo S. Morales, Jeffrey I. Algazy, Richard L. Kravitz, Michael S. Broader, David E. Kanouse, Jorge A. Muñoz, Juan-Antonio Puyol, Marielena Lara, Katherine E. Watkins, Hannah Yang, and Elizabeth A. McGlynn, "Health Information on the Internet: Accessibility, Quality, and Readability in English and Spanish," *Journal of the American Medical Association* 285, no. 20 (May 2001): 2612–2621, https://doi.org/10.1001/jama.285.20.2612.

4. Jim Giles, "Internet Encyclopaedias Go Head to Head," *Nature* 438, 900–901 (2005), https://doi.org/10.1038/438900a.

5. Adol Esquivel, Funda Meric-Bernstam, and Elmer V. Bernstam, "Accuracy and Self-Correction of Information Received from an Internet Breast Cancer List: Content Analysis," *British Medical Journal* 332, no. 7547 (April 22, 2006): 939–942, https://doi.org/10.1136/bmj.38753.524201.7C.

6. Katherine White, Amyeleh Gebremariam, Dana Lewis, Weston Nordgren, James Wedding, Josh Pasek, Ashley Garrity, Emily Hirschfeld, and Joyce M. Lee. "Motivations for Participation in an Online Social Media Community for Diabetes," *Journal of Diabetes Science and Technology* 12, no. 3 (2018): 712–718. https://doi.org/10.1177/1932296817749611.

7. Chris Allen, Ivaylo Vassilev, Anne Kennedy, and Anne Rogers. "Long-Term Condition Self-Management Support in Online Communities: A Meta-Synthesis of Qualitative Papers," *Journal of Medical Internet Research* 18, no. 3 (2016), https://doi.org/10.2196/jmir.5260.

8. Angela C. King, "Long-Term Home Mechanical Ventilation in the United States," *Respiratory Care* 57, no. 6 (June 2012): 921–32, https://doi.org/10.4187/respcare.01741.

9. Marina B. Wasilewski, Jennifer N. Stinson, and Jill I. Cameron, "Web-Based Health Interventions for Family Caregivers of Elderly Individuals: A Scoping Review," *International Journal of Medical Informatics* 103 (July 2017): 109–138, https://doi.org/10.1016/j.ijmedinf.2017.04.009.

10. Amber R. Misra, Marilyn H. Oermann, Malinda S. Teague, and Leila S. Ledbetter, "An Evaluation of Websites Offering Caregiver Education for Tracheostomy and Home Mechanical Ventilation," *Journal of Pediatric Nursing* 56 (2021): 64–69, https://doi.org/10.1016/j.pedn.2020.09.014.

11. Kate Lorig, P. D. Mazonson, and H. R. Holman, "Evidence Suggesting That Health Education for Self-Management in Patients with Chronic Arthritis Has Sustained Health Benefits While Reducing Health Care Costs," *Arthritis & Rheumatology* 36, no. 4 (1993): 439–446. https://doi.org/10.1002/art.1780360403.

12. Edwin B. Fisher, Renée I. Boothroyd, Emily A. Elstad, Laura Hays, Amy Henes, Gary R. Maslow, and Clayton Velicer, "Peer Support of Complex Health Behaviors in Prevention and Disease Management with Special Reference to Diabetes: Systematic Reviews," *Clinical Diabetes and Endocrinology* 3, no. 4 (May 25, 2017), https://doi.org/10.1186/s40842-017-0042-3.

13. Laura A. Linnan, Edwin B. Fisher, and Sula Hood, "The Power and Potential of Peer Support in Workplace Interventions," *American Journal of Health Promotion* 28, no. 1 (September 2013): 2–10, https://doi.org/10.4278/ajhp.28.1.tahp.

14. Michelle L. Litchman, Heather R. Walker, Ashley H. Ng, Sarah E. Waarzynsh, Sean M. Oser, Deborah A. Greenwood, Percy M. Gee, Mellanye Lackey, and Tamara K. Oser, "State of the Science: A Scoping Review and Gap Analysis of Diabetes Online Communities." *Journal of Diabetes Science and Technology* 13, no. 3 (May 2019): 466–492, https://doi.org/10.1177/1932296819831042.

15. Laura M. Hart, M. Teresa Granillo, Anthony F. Jorm, and Susan J. Paxton, "Unmet Need for Treatment in the Eating Disorders: A Systematic Review of Eating Disorder Specific

Treatment Seeking among Community Cases," *Clinical Psychology Review* 31, no. 5 (2011): 727–735, https://doi.org/10.1016/j.cpr.2011.03.004.

16. Dori Steinberg, Taylor Perry, David Freestone, Cara Bohon, Jessica H. Baker, and Erin Parks, "Effectiveness of Delivering Evidence-Based Eating Disorder Treatment via Telemedicine for Children, Adolescents, and Youth," *Eating Disorders*, 31, no. 1 (2022): 85–101, https://doi .org/10.1080/10640266.2022.2076334.

17. Matthew Chinman, Kevin Henze, and Patricia Sweeney, "Peer Specialist Toolkit: Implementing Peer Support Services in VHA," ed. Sharon McCarthy, *A Collaborative Project between the VISN 1 New England MIRECC Peer Education Center, and the VISN 4 MIRECC Peer Resource Center*, March 2013.

18. William H. Sledge, Martha Lawless, David Sells, Melissa Wieland, Maria J. O'Connell, and Larry Davidson, "Effectiveness of Peer Support in Reducing Readmissions of Persons with Multiple Psychiatric Hospitalizations," *Psychiatric Services* 62, no. 5 (May 2011): 541–544, https://doi.org/10.1176/ps.62.5.pss6205_0541.

19. Vikrom K. Dhar, Young Kim, Justin T. Graff, Andrew D. Jung, Jennifer Garnett, Lauren E. Dick, Jenifer Harris, and Shimul A. Shah, "Benefit of Social Media on Patient Engagement and Satisfaction: Results of a 9-Month, Qualitative Pilot Study Using Facebook," *Surgery* 163, no. 3 (March 2018): 565–570, https://doi.org/10.1016/j.surg.2017.09.056.

CHAPTER 5

1. Stav Atir, Kristina A. Wald, and Nicholas Epley, "Talking with Strangers Is Surprisingly Informative," *Proceedings of the National Academy of Sciences of the United States of America* 119, no. 34 (2022): e2206992119, https://doi.org/10.1073/pnas.2206992119.

2. Xuan Zhao and Nicholas Epley, "Surprisingly Happy to Have Helped: Underestimating Prosociality Creates a Misplaced Barrier to Asking for Help," *Psychological Science* 33, no. 10 (October 2022), https://doi.org/10.1177/09567976221097615.

3. Liz Salmi, "Spoiler Alert, I'm Still Alive: 10 Years Later," *The Liz Army* (patient blog), July 25, 2018, https://www.thelizarmy.com/blog/2018/07/spoiler-alert-im-still-alive-10-years-later.

4. Deanna J. Attai, Michael S. Cowher, Mohammed Al-Hamadani, Jody M. Schoger, Alicia C. Staley, and Jeffrey Landercasper, "Twitter Social Media Is an Effective Tool for Breast Cancer Patient Education and Support: Patient-Reported Outcomes by Survey," *Journal of Medical Internet Research* 17, no. 7 (July 2015): e188, https://doi.org/10.2196/jmir.4721.

5. Anna De Simoni, Anjali T. Shah, Olivia Fulton, Jasmine Parkinson, Aziz sheikh, Pietro Panzarasa, Claudia Pagliari, Neil S. Coulson, and Chris J. Griffiths, "Superusers' Engagement in Asthma Online Communities: Asynchronous Web-Based Interview Study," *Journal of Medical Internet Research* 22, no. 6 (2020), https://doi.org/10.2196/18185.

6. Jeffrey T. Polzer, Laurie P. Milton, and William B. Swarm Jr., "Capitalizing on Diversity: Interpersonal Congruence in Small Work Groups," *Administrative Science Quarterly* 47, no. 2 (June 2002), 296–324, https://doi.org/10.2307/3094807.

7. Matthew S. Katz, Alicia Staley, and Deanna J. Attai, "A History of #BCSM and Insights for Patient-Centered Online Interaction and Engagement," *Journal of Patient-Centered Research and Reviews* 7, no. 4 (October 2020), 304–312, https://doi.org/10.17294/2330–0698.1753.

8. Martin Roland, Sam Everington, and Martin Marshall, "Social Prescribing—Transforming the Relationship between Physicians and Their Patients," *The New England Journal of Medicine* 383, no. 2 (July 2020): 97–99, https://doi.org/10.1056/NEJMp1917060.

CHAPTER 6

1. Francesco Fornai, Patrizia Longone, Luisa Cafaro, Olga Kastsiuchenka, Michela Ferrucci, Maria Laura Manca, Gloria Lazzeri, Alida Spalloni, Natascia Bellio, Paola Lenzi, Nicola Modugno, Gabriele Siciliano, Ciro Isidoro, Luigi Murri, Stefano Ruggieri, and Antonio Paparelli, "Lithium Delays Progression of Amyotrophic Lateral Sclerosis," *Proceedings of the National Academies of Science of the United States of America* 105, no. 6 (February 2008): 2052–2057, https://doi.org/10.1073/pnas.0708022105.

2. Paul Wicks, Timothy E. Vaughan, Michael P. Massagli, and James Heywood, "Accelerated Clinical Discovery Using Self-Reported Patient Data Collected Online and a Patient-Matching Algorithm," *Nature Biotechnology* 29 (April 2011): 411–414, https://doi.org/10.1038/nbt.1837.

3. Steven Epstein, *Impure Science: AIDS, Activism, and the Politics of Knowledge* (Berkeley: University of California Press, 1996), 218–219.

4. Epstein, *Impure Science*, 286.

5. Peter Staley, "Anthony Fauci Quietly Shocked Us All," *New York Times*, December 31, 2022, https://www.nytimes.com/2022/12/31/opinion/anthony-fauci-hiv-aids-act-up.html.

6. Susannah Fox and Maeve Duggan, *Tracking for Health*, Pew Research Center, January 28, 2013, https://www.pewresearch.org/internet/2013/01/28/tracking-for-health/.

7. Jasmine Desilva, Rachel Prensky-Pomeranz, and Megan Zweig, "Digital Health Consumer Adoption Report 2020," Rock Health and the Stanford Center for Digital Health, March 1, 2021, https://rockhealth.com/reports/digital-health-consumer-adoption-report-2020/.

8. Ethan Basch, Allison M. Deal, Amylou C. Dueck, Howard I. Scher, Mark G. Kris, Clifford Hudis, and Deborah Schrag, "Overall Survival Results of a Trial Assessing Patient-Reported Outcomes for Symptom Monitoring During Routine Cancer Treatment," *Journal of the American Medical Association* 318, no. 2 (2017): 197–198, https://doi.org/10.1001/jama.2017.7156.

9. Nils B. Heyen, "From Self-Tracking to Self-Expertise: The Production of Self-Related Knowledge by Doing Personal Science," *Public Understanding of Science* 29, no. 2 (2020): 124–138, https://doi.org/10.1177/0963662519888757.

10. Gary Wolf, Thomas Blomseth Christiansen, Jacob Eg Larsen, Martijn de Groot, Steven Jonas, and Sara Riggare, *Personal Science: Learning to Observe*, LeanPub.com, 2022, last modified July 9, 2022, https://leanpub.com/Personal-Science.

11. Marcel D. Waldinger, Marcus M. H. M. Meinardi, and Dave H. Schweitzer, "Hyposensitization Therapy with Autologous Semen in Two Dutch Caucasian Males: Beneficial Effects in Postorgasmic Illness Syndrome (POIS) (Part 2)," *The Journal of Sexual Medicine* 8, no. 4 (2011): 1171–1176, https://doi.org/10.1111/j.1743–6109.2010.02167.x.

12. Anna Wexler, "Mapping the Landscape of Do-It-Yourself Medicine," *Citizen Science: Theory and Practice* 7, no. 1 (2022): 38, http://doi.org/10.5334/cstp.553.

CHAPTER 7

1. Dana M. Lewis, *Automated Insulin Delivery: How Artificial Pancreas 'Closed Loop' Systems Can Aid You in Living with Diabetes*, 2019, https://www.artificialpancreasbook.com/.

2. Dan Hurley, "Diabetes Patients Are Hacking Their Way Toward a Bionic Pancreas," *Wired*, December 24, 2014, https://www.wired.com/2014/12/diabetes-patients-hacking-together-diy-bionic-pancreases/.

CHAPTER 8

1. John A. Meyer, MD, "Werner Forssmann and Catheterization of the Heart, 1929," *Annals of Thoracic Surgery* 49, (1990): 497–499.

2. Paul van der Boor, Pedro Oliveira, and Francisco Veloso, "Users as Innovators in Developing Countries: The Global Sources of Innovation and Diffusion in Mobile Banking Services," *Research Policy* 43, no. 9 (2014): 1594–1607, https://doi.org/10.1016/j.respol.2014.05.003.

3. Harold J. Demonaco, Ayfer Ali, and Eric von Hippel, "The Major Role of Clinicians in the Discovery of Off-Label Drug Therapies," *Pharmacotherapy* 26, no. 3 (2006): 323–332, https://doi.org/10.1592/phco.26.3.323.

4. Eric von Hippel, *Free Innovation* (Cambridge MA: MIT Press, 2016), 19–25.

5. Christiana von Hippel, "A Next Generation Assets-Based Public Health Intervention Development Model: The Public as Innovators," *Frontiers in Public Health* 6, (2018): 248, https://doi.org/10.3389/fpubh.2018.00248.

6. Eric von Hippel, "Lead Users: A Source of Novel Product Concepts," *Management Science* 32 (1986): 791–805.

7. Howard Rheingold, *The Virtual Community*, electronic version, http://www.rheingold.com/vc/book/intro.html.

8. Erin Willis, "The Power of Peers: Applying User-Generated Content to Health Behaviors 'Off-Line,'" *Qualitative Health Research* 13, (November 2018): 2081–2093, https://doi.org/10.1177/1049732318786704.

9. Christoph Hienerth and Christopher Lettl, "Exploring How Peer Communities Enable Lead User Innovations to Become Standard Equipment in the Industry: Community Pull Effects," *Journal of Product Innovation Management* 28, no. 1 (November 2011): 175–195, https://doi.org/10.1111/j.1540–5885.2011.00869.x.

10. Sally Okun and Paul Wicks, "DigitalMe: A Journey towards Personalized Health and Thriving," *BioMedical Engineering OnLine* 17, no. 119 (2018), https://doi.org/10.1186/s12938-018-0553-x.

11. John Bailey and Joanna Kempner, "Standards Without Labs: Drug Development in the Psychedelic Underground," *Citizen Science: Theory and Practice* 7, no. 1 (2022): 41, http://doi.org/10.5334/cstp.527.

12. "Celebrating 3 Years of Patient Innovation: Report 2014–2017," Patient-Innovation.com, https://patient-innovation.com/sites/default/files/livro-pi-v17.pdf.

13. Pedro Oliveira, Leid Zejnilovic, Salomé Azevedo, Ana Maria Rodrigues, and Helena Canhao, "Peer Adoption and Development of Health Innovations by Patients: National Representative Study of 6204 Citizens," *Journal of Medical Internet Research* 21, no. 3 (2019), https://doi.org/10.2196/11726.

CHAPTER 9

1. Jefferson Hennesy, "The Story of the Cajun Navy: How Heroic Louisiana Volunteers Saved Thousands of Hurricane Katrina Evacuees," *The Hennessy Chronicles*, February 12, 2007, http://jeffersonhennessy.blogspot.com/2007/02/story-of-cajun-navy-how-herioc.html.

2. David Graham, "Why Ordinary Citizens Are Acting as First Responders in Houston," *The Atlantic*, August 28, 2017, https://www.theatlantic.com/politics/archive/2017/08/ordinary-citizens-are-first-responders/538233/.

3. S. Vincent Rajkumar, Susanna Jacobus, Natalie S. Callander, Rafael Fonseca, David H. Vesole, Michael E. Williams, Rafat Abonour, David S. Siegel, Michael Katz, and Philip R. Greipp, "Lenalidomide Plus High-Dose Dexamethasone versus Lenalidomide Plus Low-Dose Dexamethasone as Initial Therapy for Newly Diagnosed Multiple Myeloma: An Open-Label Randomised Controlled Trial," *The Lancet Oncology* 11, no. 1 (2010): 29–37, https://doi.org/10.1016/S1470–2045(09)70284–0.

4. Warner V. Slack, "Patient Counseling by Computer," *Proceedings of the Annual Symposium on Computer Application in Medical Care*, November 9, 1978: 222–226.

5. Warner V. Slack. "The Patient's Right to Decide," *The Lancet* 2, no. 8031 (1977): 240, https://doi.org/10.1016/s0140–6736(77)92849–5.

6. Kate R. Lorig, Deborah Lubeck, R. Guy Kraines, Mitchell, Seleznick, and Halstad R. Holman, "Outcomes of Self-Help Education for Patients with Arthritis," *Arthritis & Rheumatology* 28, no. 6 (1985): 680–685, https://doi.org/10.1002/art.1780280612.

7. Kate R. Lorig, Lisa Konkol, and Virginia Gonzalez, "Arthritis Patient Education: A Review of the Literature." *Patient Education and Counseling* 10, no. 3 (1987): 207–52, https://doi.org/10.1016/0738–3991(87)90126–1.

8. Amy Tenderich, "An Open Letter to Steve Jobs," *DiabetesMine* (blog), https://www.healthline.com/health/diabetesmine/innovation/open-letter-steve-jobs.

9. Joyce M. Lee, Emily Hirschfeld, and James Wedding, "A Patient-Designed Do-It-Yourself Mobile Technology System for Diabetes: Promise and Challenges for a New Era in Medicine," *Journal of the American Medical Association* 315, no. 14 (2016): 1447–1448, https://doi.org/10.1001/jama.2016.1903.

CHAPTER 10

1. Eliot Marshall, "Breast Cancer's Forced March?: By a Fluke of Politics, the Army Has Become the Lead Federal Agency in Breast Cancer Research; Now There Is a Tussle over How It Should Spend a $210 Million Bonanza," *Science* 258, no. 5083 (October 30, 1992): 732, https://doi.org/10.1126/science.1439774.

2. Daniel Sarewitz, "Saving Science," *The New Atlantis*, no. 49 (2016): 4–40.

3. Caroline S. Bennette, Scott D. Ramsey, Carl L. Mcdermott, Josh J. Carlson, Anirban Basu, and David L. Veenstra, "Predicting Low Accrual in the National Cancer Institute's Cooperative Group Clinical Trials," *JNCI: Journal of the National Cancer Institute*, 108, no. 2 (February 2016), https://doi.org/10.1093/jnci/djv324.

4. See, for example, Sherry Arnstein, "A Ladder of Citizen Participation," *Journal of the American Planning Association* 35, no. 4, (1969): 216–224; "Building Effective Multi-Stakeholder Research Teams," Patient-Centered Outcomes Research Institute, September 16, 2020, https://www.pcori.org/events/2020/building-effective-multi-stakeholder-research-teams; "You Need to Ask Patients: A Step-by-Step Guide to Creating a Mindset of Inclusion," Savvy Cooperative ebook, https://www.savvy.coop; "A Research Partnership Maturity Model for Patient Organizations," FasterCures, 2021, https://milkeninstitute.org/article/RPMM-companion-guide; "Patient-Led Research Scorecards," Patient-Led Research Collaborative and the Council of Medical Specialty Societies, 2023, https://cmss.org/wp-content/uploads/2023/01/11231_CMSS_Plybk_Scorecards_FINAL.pdf.

5. Andrea Wiggins and John Wilbanks, "The Rise of Citizen Science in Health and Biomedical Research," *The American Journal of Bioethics*, 19, no. 8 (2019): 3–14, https://doi.org/10.1080/15265161.2019.1619859.

6. David B. Fogel, "Factors Associated with Clinical Trials That Fail and Opportunities for Improving the Likelihood of Success: A Review," *Contemporary Clinical Trials Communications* 11 (August 2018): 156–164, https://doi.org/10.1016/j.conctc.2018.08.001.

7. Bennett Levitan, Kenneth Getz, Eric L. Eisenstein, Michelle Goldberg, Matthew Harker, Sharon Hesterlee, Bray Patrick-Lake, Jamie N. Roberts, and Joseph DiMasi, "Assessing the Financial Value of Patient Engagement: A Quantitative Approach from CTTI's Patient Groups and Clinical Trials Project," *Therapeutic Innovation & Regulatory Science* 52 (2018): 220–229. https://doi.org/10.1177/2168479017716715.

8. Philip Bradonjic, Nikolaus Franke, and Christian Lüthje, "Decision-Makers' Underestimation of User Innovation," *Research Policy* 48 (2019), https://doi.org/10.1016/j.respol.2019.01.020.

9. Ben Eloff, John Sedor, and Molly O'Neill, "Putting the Public in Public Health: KidneyX COVID-19 Kidney Care Challenge Winners," HHS.gov (blog), May 6, 2021.

10. Christoph Hienerth and Christopher Lettl, "Exploring How Peer Communities Enable Lead User Innovations to Become Standard Equipment in the Industry: Community Pull Effects," *Journal of Product Innovation Management* 28, no. 1 (November 2011): 175–195, https://doi .org/10.1111/j.1540-5885.2011.00869.x.

11. Dana Lewis, "Barriers to Citizen Science and Dissemination of Knowledge in Healthcare," *Citizen Science: Theory and Practice* 7, no. 1 (2022): 40, https://doi.org/10.5334/cstp.511.

12. Lisa D. Cook, "The Innovation Gap in Pink and Black," in *Does America Need More Innovators?*, eds. Matthew Wisnioski, Eric S. Hintz, and Marie Stettler Kleine (Cambridge, MA: MIT Press, 2019): 221–247.

CHAPTER 11

1. Paul Wicks, Dorothy L. Keininger, Michael P. Massagli, Christine de la Loge, Catherine Brownstein, Jouko Isojärvi, and James Heywood, "Perceived Benefits of Sharing Health Data between People with Epilepsy on an Online Platform," *Epilepsy & Behavior* 23, no. 1 (2012): 16–23, https://doi.org/10.1016/j.yebeh.2011.09.026.

2. Courtney R. Lyles, Urmimala Sarkar, Urvashi Patel, Sarah Lisker, Allison Stark, Vanessa Guzman, and Ashwin Patel, "Real-World Insights from Launching Remote Peer-to-Peer Mentoring in a Safety Net Healthcare Delivery Setting," *Journal of the American Medical Informatics Association* 28, no. 2 (2021): 365–370, https://doi.org/10.1093/jamia/ocaa251.

Index